I dedicate this book to all who are powerful in spirit and do not fear

CONTENTS

INTRODUCTION

The number of diseases plaguing our society is huge. There are pharmacies at every intersection. More and more people get sick, and sometimes very seriously. Most people die of diseases related to the circulatory system. Cancer is another extremely important problem. We also have a coronavirus that the world is not coping with. In addition, over 100 million adults suffer from diabetes or prediabetes in the US. Most people, including doctors, have no idea of any kind of prevention. How many of us have a family member suffering from cancer or diabetes? Probably many. Is it possible to significantly reduce the risk of developing these and other diseases? Many of the scientific publications on which this book is based indicate just that.

The information in this book is useful and valuable not only for those who want to take care of their health or regain their health, but also for doctors who want to heal more effectively. The book is based on dozens of scientific publications and long medical practice. Many of these facts are unknown at all. Many of these facts also appear to negate common recommendations. And ignorance of these facts results in the fact that many people get sick and many, unfortunately, die. The book is short but succinct and essential. The aim of the author was to reveal the functions and effects of individual vitamins and minerals in such a way that the book was readable for an ordinary person who is not interested in reading long stories but also a contribution to further investigation for doctors.

This is not a novel, but a collection of huge amounts of crucial, often hidden facts. Every household should have at least one copy of this book and use the knowledge contained in it to stay healthy.

This book is not a medical textbook. You have to remember that each organism is different and reacts differently to different substances. The book is a collection of information, not advice. Before using any substance, you should consult a doctor.

BRIEFLY ABOUT THE BODY'S IMMUNITY...

The immune system is very complex and involves thousands of substances such as enzymes, hormones and acids. Our body always strives for homeostasis, i.e. the biological balance of the body. For this, the body needs many substances, including vitamins and minerals. The organism cannot be also exposed to substances the action of which prevents the organism from achieving homeostasis. Such substances include, for example, heavy metals, pesticides and various types of drugs. Many of them lead to the so-called oxidative stress. Oxidative stress can also be caused by ionizing radiation, toxins contained in cigarette smoke or various pathogens.

When one electron is detached from an oxygen molecule, a free radical is formed. A free radical is a molecular species that contains an unpaired electron in an atomic orbital. This is the case not only with oxygen but also with nitrogen. When our antioxidant system cannot cope with a large number of free radicals, free radicals take away the missing electron from other atoms, and these atoms take electrons from the next atoms again. There are many types of free radicals. A large number of oxidative reactions have a very negative effect on our body.

On the other hand, antioxidants are substances that give up one electron and then also become free radicals. But not harmful to the body.

Too many oxidative reactions in the body is called oxidative stress. This is the beginning of many diseases and a huge problem for the body. Free radicals contribute greatly to cancer, rheumatoid arthritis, Alzheimer's, diabetes, multiple sclerosis, Crohn's disease, asthma, arteriosclerosis and much more. Many specialists believe that free radicals are the cause of all diseases...

A few more words...

First it must be said that vitamins and minerals should be absorbed from food. Vitamin C, for example, from vegetables or fruit, along with thousands of other substances, is not the same as ascorbic acid itself. It should be so, but is it so? As we know, the quality of food in the United States or Europe is almost tragic. What if we also have problems absorbing this poor food because of problems with the functioning of the stomach or intestines? **You are not what you eat but what you absorb!** Often, in many cases, supplementation is inevitable. In case of ailments, a normal diet may not be enough. And as research and medical practice show, many supposedly incurable diseases turn out to be curable.

VITAMIN D

Research shows that vitamin D receptors are found on every human cell. Who knows about this at all, except the readers of this book now?

Vitamin D3 or as some say D3 hormone should be the first thing in the treatment and prevention of autoimmune diseases. Dr. Cedric Garland, based on many years of research, concluded that the level of vitamin D should be at least 60 ng / ml. He also concluded that if vitamin D levels were adequate, the incidence of breast cancer, colorectal cancer, kidney cancer and multiple sclerosis would be reduced by as much as 50 to 80%. That's quite a lot...

Dr. Bruce Hollis, author of over 200 scientific publications, states that blood levels of vitamin D below 32 ng / ml should be considered as deficiency.

When vitamin D levels are high, the body produces certain protein complexes that are highly bactericidal and virucidal. Maybe vitamin D would also have a significant effect on Covid-19? It turns out that it does.

Gröber U, Holick MF. The coronavirus disease (COVID-19) - **A supportive approach with selected**

micronutrients. Int J Vitam Nutr Res. 2021 Jan 25:1-22. doi: 10.1024/0300-9831/a000693. Epub ahead of print. PMID: 33487035.

For 191,779 patients in 50 US states, Sars-CoV-2 positives rates were inversely related to vitamin D levels. In other words, you are much more likely to get the disease if you have low levels of vitamin D.

"For the entire population those who had a circulating level of 25(OH)D < 20 ng/mL had a 54% higher positivity rate compared to those who had a blood level of 30–34 ng/mL. The risk for SARS-CoV-2 infection continued to decline until the serum levels reached 55 ng/mL."

Lakkireddy, M., Gadiga, S.G., Malathi, R.D. et al. **Impact of daily high dose oral vitamin D therapy on the inflammatory markers in patients with COVID 19 disease.** Sci Rep 11, 10641 (2021). https://doi.org/10.1038/s41598-021-90189-4

The study looked at Impact of daily high dose oral vitamin D therapy on the inflammatory markers (N / L ratio, CRP, LDH, IL6, Ferritin) in patients with COVID 19 disease. Patients were divided into two groups. The first one got 60,000 IUs of vitamin D daily for 8 or 10 days depending upon their BMI in addition to the standard treatment. The second group received standard treatment alone. In the first group, a very significant decrease in all measured markers of inflammation was noted. The reduction of markers in the second group was insignificant. Researchers indicated that therapeutic improvement of vitamin D levels to 80-100 ng / ml significantly reduced the markers of inflammation associated with COVID-19 without any side effects, and the vitamin itself could prove very helpful in therapy.

Jain, A., Chaurasia, R., Sengar, N.S. et al. **Analysis of vitamin D level among asymptomatic and critically ill COVID-19 patients and its correlation with inflammatory markers.** Sci Rep 10, 20191 (2020). https://doi.org/10.1038/s41598-020-77093-z

In another study out of 154 patients 91 were asymptomatic (Group A). 63 patients were severely ill and had required ICU admission (Group B). The prevalence of vitamin D deficiency was 31.86% in Group A. In Group B 96.82% patients were vitamin D deficient.

The authors of other studies conclude: "Vitamin D deficiency markedly increases the chance of having severe disease after infection with SARS Cov-2. The intensity of inflammatory response is also higher in vitamin D deficient COVID-19 patients. This all translates to increase morbidity and mortality in COVID-19 patients who are deficient in vitamin D.

Keeping the current COVID-19 pandemic in view authors recommend administration of vitamin D supplements to population at risk for COVID-19."

Urashima M, Segawa T, Okazaki M, Kurihara M, Wada Y, Ida H. **Randomized trial of vitamin D supplementation to prevent seasonal influenza A in schoolchildren.** Am J Clin Nutr. 2010 May;91(5):1255-60. doi: 10.3945/ajcn.2009.29094. Epub 2010 Mar 10. PMID: 20219962.

"This study suggests that vitamin D (3) supplementation during the winter may reduce the incidence of influenza A, especially in specific subgroups of schoolchildren".

Vitamin D reduces the risk of getting seasonal influenza. I know also from my own experience that people who have the right level of vitamin D3 do not get seasonal flu.

Vitamin D is a very important component in the prevention of cancer.

Robien K, Cutler GJ, Lazovich D. **Vitamin D intake and breast in postmenopausal women: the Iowa Women's Health Study**. Cancer Causes Control.2007 Sep;18(7):775-82. doi: 10.1007/s10552-007-9020-x. Epub 2007 Jun 5. PMID: 17549593.

Garland CF, Garland FC, Gorham ED, et al. **The role of vitamin D in cancer prevention.** Am J Public Health. 2006;96(2):252-261. doi:10.2105/AJPH.2004.045260

Adequately high vitamin D levels significantly reduce cancer incidence.

Chandler PD, Chen WY, Ajala ON, Hazra A, Cook N, Bubes V, Lee IM, Giovannucci EL, Willett W, Buring JE, Manson JE; VITAL Research Group. **Effect of Vitamin D3 Supplements on Development of Advanced Cancer: A Secondary Analysis of the VITAL Randomized Clinical Trial.** JAMA Netw Open. 2020 Nov 2;3(11):e2025850. doi: 10.1001/jamanetworkopen.2020.25850. Erratum in: JAMA Netw Open. 2020 Dec 1;3(12):e2032460. PMID: 33206192; PMCID: PMC7675103.

Scientists from Harvard Medical School have also shown that vitamin D supplementation reduced the incidence of advanced (metastatic or fatal) cancer.

Yuan C, Sato K, Hollis BW, Zhang S, Niedzwiecki D, Ou FS, Chang IW, O'Neil BH, Innocenti F, Lenz HJ, Blanke CD, Goldberg RM,

Venook AP, Mayer RJ, Fuchs CS, Meyerhardt JA, Ng K. **Plasma 25-Hydroxyvitamin D Levels and Survival in Patients with Advanced or Metastatic Colorectal Cancer**: Findings from CALGB/SWOG 80405 (Alliance). Clin Cancer Res. 2019 Dec 15;25(24):7497-7505. doi: 10.1158/1078-0432.CCR-19-0877. Epub 2019 Sep 23. PMID: 31548349; PMCID: PMC6911644.

Higher levels of vitamin D had a positive effect on patients with advanced or metastatic colorectal cancer. Interestingly, 63% of patients had vitamin d levels < 20 ng / mL and 31% had levels 20- < 30 ng / mL.

Madden JM, Murphy L, Zgaga L, Bennett K. **De novo vitamin D supplement use post-diagnosis is associated with breast cancer survival.** Breast Cancer Res Treat. 2018 Nov;172(1):179-190. doi: 10.1007/s10549-018-4896-6. Epub 2018 Jul 23. PMID: 30039288.

In a study of 5,417 women with a record of invasive breast cancer aged 50-80 years, 2,581 women were administered vitamin D. If vitamin D was initiated soon after the breast cancer diagnosis (within 6 months) there was a 49% reduction in mortality.

Ekmekcioglu C, Haluza D, Kundi M. **25-Hydroxy-**

vitamin D Status and Risk for Colorectal Cancer and Type 2 Diabetes Mellitus: A Systematic Review and Meta-Analysis of Epidemiological Studies. Int J Environ Res Public Health. 2017 Jan 28;14(2):127. doi: 10.3390/ijerph14020127. PMID: 28134804; PMCID: PMC5334681.

Mata-analysis showed a 39% risk reduction for colorectal cancer when comparing individuals with the highest category of 25 (OH) D with those in the lowest.

Amaral AF, Méndez-Pertuz M, Muñoz A, Silverman DT, Allory Y, Kogevinas M, Lloreta J, Rothman N, Carrato A, Rivas del Fresno M, Real FX, Malats N; Spanish Bladder Cancer/EPICURO Study investigators. **Plasma 25-hydroxyvitamin D(3) and bladder cancer risk according to tumor stage and FGFR3 status:** a mechanism-based epidemiological study. J Natl Cancer Inst. 2012 Dec 19;104(24):1897-904. doi: 10.1093/jnci/djs444. Epub 2012 Oct 29. PMID: 23108201; PMCID: PMC3525815.

Another study found that the risk of carcinoma doubles if the vitamin D level is low. The relationship is especially strong in patients with muscle-invasive tumors.

Munger KL, Levin LI, Hollis BW, Howard NS,

Ascherio A. **Serum 25-hydroxyvitamin D levels and risk of multiple sclerosis.** JAMA. 2006 Dec 20;296(23):2832-8. doi: 10.1001/jama.296.2-3.2832. PMID: 17179460.

Ramagopalan SV, Maugeri NJ, Handunnetthi L, Lincoln MR, Orton SM, Dyment DA, Deluca GC, Herrera BM, Chao MJ, Sadovnick AD, Ebers GC, Knight JC. **Expression of the multiple sclerosis-associated MHC class II Allele HLA-DRB1*1501 is regulated by vitamin D.** PLoS Genet. 2009 Feb;5(2):e1000369. doi: 10.1371/journal.pgen.1000369. Epub 2009 Feb 6. PMID: 19197344; PMCID: PMC2627899.

Research shows that the risk of developing multiple sclerosis can be reduced as long as the vitamin D level is adequate.

Hyppönen E, Läärä E, Reunanen A, Järvelin MR, Virtanen SM. **Intake of vitamin D and risk of type 1 diabetes: a birth-cohort study.** Lancet. 2001 Nov 3;358(9292):1500-3. doi: 10.1016/S0140-6736(01)06580-1. PMID: 11705562.

Additionally: "Dietary vitamin D supplementation is associated with reduced risk of type 1 diabetes. Ensuring adequate vitamin D supplementation for infants could help to reverse the increasing trend in

the incidence of type 1 diabetes".
Risk can be reduced by up to 88%.

Farnik H, Bojunga J, Berger A, Allwinn R, Waidmann O, Kronenberger B, Keppler OT, Zeuzem S, Sarrazin C, Lange CM. **Low vitamin D serum concentration is associated with high levels of hepatitis B virus replication in chronically infected patients.** Hepatology. 2013 Oct;58(4):1270-6. doi: 10.1002/hep.26488. Epub 2013 Aug 7. PMID: 23703797.

In addition: "Low 25(OH)D3 serum levels are associated with high levels of HBV (hepatitis B virus) replication in patients with CHB (chronic hepatitis B)".
This is important information regarding the effects of vitamin D on the development of the hepatitis B virus for patients with this disease. Now is just time to try.

Vitamin D is involved in the functioning of bone-building minerals and it helps to maintain the balance between calcium and phosphorus in the body.

Anderson PH, Lam NN, Turner AG, Davey RA, Kogawa M, Atkins GJ, Morris HA. **The pleiotropic effects of vitamin D in bone.** J Steroid Biochem Mol Biol. 2013 Jul;136:190-4. doi: 10.1016/j.jsbmb.2012.08.008. Epub 2012 Sep 5. PMID: 22981997.

It inhibits excessive bone degradation.

DeLuca HF. **Overview of general physiologic features and functions of vitamin D.** Am J Clin Nutr. 2004 Dec;80(6 Suppl):1689S-96S. doi: 10.1093/ajcn/80.6.1689S. PMID: 15585789.

"The hormonal form of vitamin D3, ie, 1α, 25-dihydroxyvitamin D3, acts through a nuclear receptor to carry out its many functions, including calcium absorption, phosphate absorption in the intestine, calcium mobilization in bone, and calcium reabsorption in the kidney. It also has several noncalcemic functions in the body."

It promotes the absorption of calcium and phosphorus from the intestines, the reabsorption of calcium in the kidneys and the incorporation of calcium into the bones. Vitamin D also regulates the action of osteoblasts.

Peppone LJ, Hebl S, Purnell JQ, Reid ME, Rosier RN, Mustian KM, Palesh OG, Huston AJ, Ling MN, Morrow GR. **The efficacy of calcitriol therapy in the management of bone loss and fractures: a qualitative review.** Osteoporos Int. 2010 Jul;21(7):1133-49. doi: 10.1007/s00198-009-1136-2. Epub 2009 Dec 4. PMID: 19960185; PMCID: PMC3063996.

Vitamin D in the active form of calcitriol is effective in the treatment of osteoporosis. Low blood levels of vitamin D are also associated with lower bone mineral density, which increases the risk of bone fracture.

Chapuy MC, Arlot ME, Duboeuf F, Brun J, Crouzet B, Arnaud S, Delmas PD, Meunier PJ. **Vitamin D3 and calcium to prevent hip fractures in elderly women.** N Engl J Med. 1992 Dec 3;327(23):1637-42. doi: 10.1056/NEJM199212033272305. PMID: 1331788.

In elderly women who have been given 1,200 mg of calcium and 800 units of vitamin D3 daily for 18 months: "Among the women who completed the 18-month study, the number of hip fractures was 43 percent lower (P = 0.043) and the total number of nonvertebral fractures was 32 percent lower (P = 0.015) among the women treated with vitamin D3 and calcium than among those who received placebo".

Ostadmohammadi V, Jamilian M, Bahmani F, Asemi Z. **Vitamin D and probiotic co-supplementation** affects mental health, hormonal, inflammatory and oxidative stress parameters in women with polycystic ovary syndrome. J Ovarian Res. 2019 Jan 21;12(1):5. doi: 10.1186/s13048-019-0480-x. PMID: 30665436; PMCID: PMC6340184.

Vitamin D with probiotics had beneficial effects on mental health parameters, serum total testosterone, hirsutism in women with polycystic ovary syndrome (PCOS).

Akbari M, Ostadmohammadi V, Lankarani KB, Tabrizi R, Kolahdooz F, Heydari ST, Kavari SH, Mirhosseini N, Mafi A, Dastorani M, Asemi Z. **The Effects of Vitamin D Supplementation on Biomarkers of Inflammation and Oxidative Stress Among Women with Polycystic Ovary Syndrome**: A Systematic Review and Meta-Analysis of Randomized Controlled Trials. Horm Metab Res. 2018 Apr;50(4):271-279. doi: 10.1055/s-0044-101355. Epub 2018 Feb 23. PMID: 29475212.

Vitamin D had also a beneficial effect on inflammation and oxidative stress in women with polycystic ovary syndrome.

This vitamin may also be helpful in treating rheumatoid arthritis. The improvement is related to the reduction of inflammation. The risk of other ailments associated with this disease is also reduced.

Vitamin D deficiency is associated with underdevelopment of the pelvis in young girls, which in the future may result in not having a child naturally due to too small pelvic bones.

Merewood A, Mehta SD, Chen TC, Bauchner H, Holick MF. **Association between vitamin D deficiency and primary cesarean section.** J Clin Endocrinol Metab. 2009;94(3):940-945. doi:1-0.1210/jc.2008-1217

In a study of 400 pregnant women, women with adequate vitamin D levels had a four times lower risk of having surgery in childbirth.

According to Dr. Hollis, about 10% of the mother's vitamin D will go into her milk. For example, a mother, taking 5,000 IU / day, will give her child about 500 IU / liter in milk. Once the mother is getting enough vitamin D, there is no need to artificially give this vitamin to the newborn.

Vitamin D can help with depression. I know from experience that the well-being improves significantly in the range of 100-150 ng / ml.

Vitamin D levels (i.e. Metabolite 25(OH)D) should be measured from time to time. The best source of vitamin D is the sun. UVB is the only fraction of sunlight that enables production of vitamin D. However, it is not about long sunbathing. We should do it briefly, e.g. when in a swimsuit, the front of the body for 15 minutes and the back for 15 minutes. We do it when the sun is highest, that is, the angle of the sun's rays is highest. The closer to the equator, the easier it will be to take care of vitamin D (although it also depends on skin color and weather). Here in Paris, it is possible to use the sun to produce vitamin D from around April to September. It is best to do it between 11:00 a.m. and 1 p.m. It will be different in the US or UK.

Long exposure to the sun can lead to skin cancer, but a short midday sun exposure is very beneficial for us. Older adults have a harder time producing vitamin D from the sun. And what if I can't enjoy the sun? How much should I take this vitamin D3? Of course, this cannot be easily stated. It all depends on what level of vitamin D we have in our blood and what we would like to have. Different levels of this vitamin are sufficient for effective prevention and different levels for serious treatment. Sometimes we only need 5000-10000 IU / day to maintain our level. If our vitamin D level is low, it may be 15,000 IU to 25,000 IU per day to raise this level, and in the case of treatment (e.g. cancer), 50,000 IU or even 100,000 IU / day. It is difficult to overdose on vitamin D. It is best to supplement vitamin D with other fat-soluble vitamins (mainly vitamin K2). Magnesium and boron is also crucial.

VITAMIN K2

Vitamin K2 helps transport electrons in the mitochondria and produce energy. It controls where calcium builds up in the body. Vitamin K2 prevents calcium from accumulating in the inappropriate places, especially in soft tissues and arteries. Vitamin K2 does this by increasing the production of MGP (Matrix GLA Protein), which regulates calcium in the body.

Flore R, Ponziani FR, Di Rienzo TA, Zocco MA, Flex A, Gerardino L, Lupascu A, Santoro L, Santoliquido A, Di Stasio E, Chierici E, Lanti A, Tondi P, Gasbarrini A. **Something more to say about calcium homeostasis: the role of vitamin K2 in vascular calcification and osteoporosis**. Eur Rev Med Pharmacol Sci. 2013 Sep;17(18):2433-40. PMID: 24089220.

"Vitamin K2 deficiency has recently been recognized as a protagonist in the development of vascular calcification and osteoporosis. Data reported so far are promising and dietary supplementation seems a useful tool to contrast these diseases".

For this reason, it has a positive effect on bones and

the heart.

Maresz K. Proper **Calcium Use: Vitamin K2 as a Promoter of Bone and Cardiovascular Health**. Integr Med (Encinitas). 2015;14(1):34-39.

Vitamin K2 is associated with the inhibition of arterial calcification. Adequate intake of vitamin K2 reduces the risk of vascular damage as it activates the matrix GLA protein, which inhibits calcium deposition on the artery walls. In other words, if you lack vitamin K2, your bones fail to take in calcium and it begins to build up in your arteries. Therefore, large amounts of calcium and vitamin D without K2 can be dangerous.

Iwamoto J, Takeda T, Sato Y. **Effects of vitamin K2 on osteoporosis**. Curr Pharm Des. 2004;10(21):2557-76. doi: 10.2174/1381612043383782. PMID: 15320745.

Studies have shown that vitamin K2 may be useful in preventing or treating fractures, osteoporosis, and osteomalacia. In addition, clinical studies have shown that K2 slows the rate of bone loss in adults.

Kaneki M. [**Vitamin K2 as a protector of bone health and beyond**]. Clin Calcium. 2005

Apr;15(4):605-10. Japanese. PMID: 15802772.

People with osteoporosis who supplement vitamin K2 have significantly fewer bone fractures than people without supplementation.

Kaneki M, Hodges SJ, Hosoi T, Fujiwara S, Lyons A, Crean SJ, Ishida N, Nakagawa M, Takechi M, Sano Y, Mizuno Y, Hoshino S, Miyao M, Inoue S, Horiki K, Shiraki M, Ouchi Y, Orimo H. **Japanese fermented soybean food as the major determinant of the large geographic difference in circulating levels of vitamin K2: possible implications for hip-fracture risk.** Nutrition. 2001 Apr;17(4):315-21. doi: 10.1016/s0899-9007(00)00554-2. Erratum in: Nutrition. 2006 Oct;22(10):1075. Hedges, S J [corrected to Hodges, S J]. PMID: 11369171.

"These findings indicate that the large geographic difference in MK-7 levels may be ascribed, at least in part, to natto intake and suggest the possibility that higher MK-7 level resulting from natto consumption may contribute to the relatively lower fracture risk in Japanese women".

Vitamin K2 also supports proper dentition.

Especially vitamin K2 MK-7 can protect against

ischemic heart disease.

Geleijnse JM, Vermeer C, Grobbee DE, Schurgers LJ, Knapen MH, van der Meer IM, Hofman A, Witteman JC. **Dietary intake of menaquinone is associated with a reduced risk of coronary heart disease: the Rotterdam Study.** J Nutr. 2004 Nov;134(11):3100-5. doi: 10.1093/jn/134.11.3100. PMID: 15514282.

After supplementation with vitamin K2, there was a lower risk of aortic calcification in a study of 4,807 people. Individuals had a 52% lower risk of severe aortic calcification and a 41% lower risk of coronary heart disease.
Why is it so little talked about when it is one of the most serious health problems in our society?

Bolland MJ, Grey A, Avenell A, Gamble GD, Reid IR. **Calcium supplements with or without vitamin D and risk of cardiovascular events: re-analysis of the Women's Health Initiative limited access dataset and meta-analysis.** BMJ. 2011 Apr 19;342:d2040. doi: 10.1136/bmj.d2040. PMID: 21505219; PMCID: PMC3079822.

Bolland MJ, Barber PA, Doughty RN, Mason B, Horne A, Ames R, Gamble GD, Grey A, Reid IR. **Vascular events in healthy older women rece-**

iving calcium supplementation: randomised controlled trial. BMJ. 2008 Feb 2;336(7638):262-6. doi: 10.1136/bmj.39440.525752.BE. Epub 2008 Jan 15. PMID: 18198394; PMCID: PMC2222999.

Women who took calcium supplements to prevent osteoporosis were more likely to develop arterial calcification, heart attack and stroke. And don't they honk everywhere to take calcium? Anyone know what are the risks of calcium supplementation alone? Readers of this book do. This is where vitamin K2 is essential.

Zwakenberg SR, Burgess S, Sluijs I, Weiderpass E; EPIC-CVD consortium, Beulens JWJ, van der Schouw YT. **Circulating phylloquinone, inactive Matrix Gla protein and coronary heart disease risk: A two-sample Mendelian Randomization study.** ClinNutr.2020Apr;39(4):1131-1136.doi: 10.1016/j.clnu.2019.04.024. Epub 2019 May 7. PMID: 31103344.

"However, lower dp-ucMGP levels may be causally related with a decreased CHD risk".

Gast GC, de Roos NM, Sluijs I, Bots ML, Beulens JW, Geleijnse JM, Witteman JC, Grobbee DE, Peeters PH, van der Schouw YT. **A high menaquinone intake reduces the incidence of coronary heart disease.**

Nutr Metab Cardiovasc Dis. 2009 Sep;19(7):504-10. doi: 10.1016/j.numecd.2008.10.004. Epub 2009 Jan 28. PMID: 19179058.

"A high intake of menaquinones, especially MK-7, MK-8 and MK-9, could protect against CHD".

A high intake of K2 protected against arterial calcification and heart disease. Examples of such publications could be mentioned and mentioned...

Lee NK, Sowa H, Hinoi E, Ferron M, Ahn JD, Confavreux C, Dacquin R, Mee PJ, McKee MD, Jung DY, Zhang Z, Kim JK, Mauvais-Jarvis F, Ducy P, Karsenty G. **Endocrine regulation of energy metabolism by the skeleton.** Cell. 2007 Aug 10;130(3):456-69. doi: 10.1016/j.cell.2007.05.047. PMID: 17693256; PMCID: PMC2013746.

Vitamin K2 may be useful in treating type 2 diabetes. Osteocalcin, which under the influence of vitamin K2 is stimulated, influences the sensitization of cells to the action of insulin.

Sakamoto N, Nishiike T, Iguchi H, Sakamoto K. **Relationship between acute insulin response and vitamin K intake in healthy young male volunteers.** Diabetes Nutr Metab. 1999 Feb;12(1):37-41. PMID: 10517305.

"Insulinogenic index (incremental IRI/incremental PG, 0-30 min) of the low VK intake group was significantly lower than that of the high intake group (0.4 vs 0.9). These results suggested that VK (Vitamin K2) may play an important role on the acute insulin response in glucose tolerance".

The positive effect of vitamin K2 on glucose tolerance was also demonstrated in the study with 25 healthy young male volunteers.

Sakamoto N, Nishiike T, Iguchi H, Sakamoto K. **Possible effects of one week vitamin K (menaquinone-4) tablets intake on glucose tolerance in healthy young male volunteers with different descarboxy prothrombin levels.** Clin Nutr. 2000 Aug;19(4):259-63. doi: 10.1054/clnu.2000.0102. PMID: 10952797.

After one week of vitamin K2 supplementation (90 mg of menaquinone-4/d), diabetic patients reduced their post meal insulin levels by half. Thus, vitamin K2 supports the work of insulin. This knowledge might help many patients struggling with this disease. But who of them knows about it?

Schwalfenberg GK. Vitamins K1 and K2: **The Emerging Group of Vitamins Required for Human Health.** J Nutr Metab. 2017;2017:6254836. doi:

10.1155/2017/6254836. Epub 2017 Jun 18. PMID: 28698808; PMCID: PMC5494092.

"Vitamin K2 may safely suppress growth and invasion of human hepatocellular carcinoma via protein kinase A activation and result in moderate suppression of tumor recurrence. It has also been shown to result in growth suppression in a dose dependent manner in lung cancer cells in vitro. Similar results were found in pancreatic cancer cells. A cohort study (LOE = B) of over 11,000 patients showed that higher vitamin K2 intake was associated with a significant reduction in advanced prostate cancer in particular".

Vitamin K2 can help prevent certain types of cancer. This mainly applies to advanced prostate and liver cancer.

Juanola-Falgarona M, Salas-Salvadó J, Martínez-González MÁ, Corella D, Estruch R, Ros E, Fitó M, Arós F, Gómez-Gracia E, Fiol M, Lapetra J, Basora J, Lamuela-Raventós RM, Serra-Majem L, Pintó X, Muñoz MÁ, Ruiz-Gutiérrez V, Fernández-Ballart J, Bulló M. **Dietary intake of vitamin K is inversely associated with mortality risk.** J Nutr. 2014 May;144(5):743-50. doi: 10.3945/jn.113.187740. Epub 2014 Mar 19. Erratum in: J Nutr. 2016 Mar;146(3):653. PMID: 24647393.

Furthermore: "An increase in dietary intake of vitamin K is associated with a reduced risk of cardiovascular, cancer, or all-cause mortality in a Mediterranean population at high cardiovascular disease risk".

Yoshida T, Miyazawa K, Kasuga I, Yokoyama T, Minemura K, Ustumi K, Aoshima M, Ohyashiki K. **Apoptosis induction of vitamin K2 in lung carcinoma cell lines: the possibility of vitamin K2 therapy for lung cancer.** Int J Oncol. 2003 Sep;23(3):627-32. PMID: 12888897.

Vitamin K2 can help with lung cancer as it inhibits the growth of all lung cancer. It has also a positive effect on leukemia.

Shea MK, Booth SL, Massaro JM, et al. **Vitamin K and vitamin D status: associations with inflammatory markers in the Framingham Offspring Study.** Am J Epidemiol. 008;167(3):313-320. doi:10.1093/aje/kwm306

"The observation that high vitamin K status was associated with lower concentrations of inflammatory markers suggests that a protective role for vitamin K in inflammation merits further investigation".

High levels of vitamin K2 are able to reduce inflammation. And it should be remembered that almost all diseases are associated with inflammation.

Vitamin K2 is also related to the central nervous system and the brain. It can help prevent a disease such as Alzheimer's disease.

Presse N, Shatenstein B, Kergoat MJ, Ferland G. **Low vitamin K intakes in community-dwelling elders at an early stage of Alzheimer's disease.** J Am Diet Assoc. 2008 Dec;108(12):2095-9. doi: 10.1016/j.jada.2008.09.013. PMID: 19027415.

It turns out that Alzheimer's patients always have low levels of vitamin K2.

Allison AC. **The possible role of vitamin K deficiency in the pathogenesis of Alzheimer's disease and in augmenting brain damage associated with cardiovascular disease.** Med Hypotheses. 2001 Aug;57(2):151-5. doi: 10.1054/mehy.2001.1307. PMID: 11461163.

"The hypothesis is now proposed that vitamin K deficiency contributes to the pathogenesis of AD (Alzheimer's disease) and that vitamin K supplementation may have a beneficial effect in preventing or treating the disease. Vitamin K may also reduce neuronal damage associated with cardiovascular disease".

Vitamin K2 helps to control disturbed calcium regulatory processes in the brain.

Vitamin K2 may be also helpful in this disease for another reason. Because it increases the sensitivity of cells to insulin. The patient's brain cannot use glucose properly. Insulin administration improves their symptoms.

Ferland G. **Vitamin K and the nervous system: an overview of its actions.** Adv Nutr. 2012 Mar 1;3(2):204-12. doi: 10.3945/an.111.001784. PMID: 22516728; PMCID: PMC3648721.

Denisova NA, Booth SL. **Vitamin K and sphingolipid metabolism: evidence to date.** Nutr Rev. 2005 Apr;63(4):111-21. doi: 10.1111/j.1753-4887.2005.tb00129.x. PMID: 15869125.

Vitamin K2 is essential for brain health at all and has multiple different functions. Vitamin K2 deficiency is associated with abnormal sphingolipid metabolism, which is associated with neurodegenerative diseases such as Alzheimer's or Parkinson's disease.

Thijssen HH, Drittij-Reijnders MJ. **Vitamin K status**

in human tissues: tissue-specific accumulation of phylloquinone and menaquinone-4. Br J Nutr. 1996 Jan;75(1):121-7. doi: 10.1079/bjn19960115. PMID: 8785182.

It can help prevent multiple sclerosis. It contributes to the proper formation of the nerve insulating layer - myelin.

Karamali M, Ashrafi M, Razavi M, Jamilian M, Akbari M, Asemi Z. **The Effects of Calcium, Vitamins D and K co-Supplementation on Markers of Insulin Metabolism and Lipid Profiles in Vitamin D-Deficient Women with Polycystic Ovary Syndrome.** Exp Clin Endocrinol Diabetes. 2017 May;125(5):316-321. doi: 10.1055/s-0043-104530. Epub 2017 Apr 13. Erratum in: Exp Clin Endocrinol Diabetes. 2020 Nov;128(11):771. PMID: 28407660

K2 supplementation may also be beneficial for improving the health of women with polycystic ovary syndrome (PCOS).

Vitamin K2 in particular, along with other fat-soluble vitamins, can help with rheumatoid arthritis. This applies to calcifications, which we can get rid of with this vitamin.

Furthermore, vitamin K2 deficiency can be one of the many causes of kidney stones.

A toxic dose for vitamin K2 has not been identified. The daily requirement of vitamin K2 in adults is about 90–120 micrograms. In the case of vitamin D3 supplementation, the dose should be increased to 200 or 300 micrograms. Vitamin K2-MK7 seems to be better than MK4 due to the longer half-life of the disintegration in the body.

High vitamin K2 foods per 100g:
- Natto - 1100µg (only MK7)
- Goose liver - 369µg (only MK4)
- Hard cheeses - 76µg (6% MK4)
- Soft cheeses - 56,5µg (6,5% MK4)
- Egg yolk - 32µg (98% MK4)
- Butter - 15µg (Only MK4)
- Chicken liver - 14µg (only MK4)
- Chicken meat - 9µg (only MK4)

VITAMIN A

Vitamin A is retinol, which is actually made up of three substances called retinoids. Beta-carotene is not vitamin A. It's a provitamin. Vitamin A is produced by the liver after the absorption of beta-carotene. If someone says that, for example, there is vitamin A in carrots, that person is wrong. However, there are more problems with beta-carotene...

Novotny JA, Harrison DJ, Pawlosky R, Flanagan VP, Harrison EH, Kurilich AC. **Beta-carotene conversion to vitamin A decreases as the dietary dose increases in humans.** J Nutr. 2010 May;140(5):915-8. doi: 10.3945/jn.109.116947. Epub 2010 Mar 17. PMID: 20237064; PMCID: PMC2855261.

"These results establish that, in humans, beta-carotene conversion to vitamin A decreases as the dietary dose increases."
Beta-carotene is absorbed only in 20–50% and the more we consume it, the lower its absorption. It should also be consumed with fat. In addition, when absorbed from one unit of beta-carotene, the body produces only 1/6 to 1/48 of unit vitamin A.

So drinking liters of carrot juice to ensure you get enough vitamin A may not be the best solution.

Vitamin A has anti-cancer and antioxidant properties. So it fights free radicals that nobody would like to have in excess.

Formelli F, Meneghini E, Cavadini E, Camerini T, Di Mauro MG, De Palo G, Veronesi U, Berrino F, Micheli A. **Plasma retinol and prognosis of postmenopausal breast cancer patients.** Cancer Epidemiol Biomarkers Prev. 2009 Jan;18(1):42-8. doi: 10.1158/1055-9965.EPI-08-0496. PMID: 19124479.

"Low plasma retinol strongly predicts poorer prognosis in postmenopausal breast cancer patients. Retinol levels should be determined as part of the prognostic workup."

Pastorino U, Infante M, Maioli M, Chiesa G, Buyse M, Firket P, Rosmentz N, Clerici M, Soresi E, Valente M, et al. **Adjuvant treatment of stage I lung cancer with high-dose vitamin A.** J Clin Oncol. 1993 Jul;11(7):1216-22. doi: 10.1200/JCO.1993.11.7.1216. PMID: 8391063.

Furthermore: "Daily oral administration of high-dose vitamin A is effective in reducing the number of new primary tumors related to tobacco consumption and may improve the disease-free interval in patients curatively resected for stage I lung cancer".

Schenk JM, Riboli E, Chatterjee N, Leitzmann MF, Ahn J, Albanes D, Reding DJ, Wang Y, Friesen MD, Hayes RB, Peters U. **Serum retinol and prostate cancer risk: a nested case-control study in the prostate, lung, colorectal, and ovarian cancer screening trial.** Cancer Epidemiol Biomarkers Prev. 2009 Apr;18(4):1227-31. doi: 10.1158/1055-9965.EPI-08-0984. Epub 2009 Mar 31. PMID: 19336558; PMCID: PMC2717001.

And: "Our results suggest that higher circulating concentrations of retinol are associated with a decreased risk of aggressive prostate cancer".
Vitamin A affects the proper functioning of the immune system.

Pinnock CB, Douglas RM, Badcock NR. **Vitamin A status in children who are prone to respiratory tract infections.** Aust Paediatr J. 1986 May;22(2):95-9. doi: 10.1111/j.1440-1754.1986.tb00197.x. PMID: 3524531.

Children who received 450 micrograms/day of vitamin A suffered from respiratory illnesses much less frequently. Grandparents always ate the liver at least once a week. Why aren't kids now given liver, which is also incredibly rich in other nutrients, and instead given carrot juices full of sugar from the store?

Farhangi MA, Keshavarz SA, Eshraghian M, Ostadrahimi A, Saboor-Yaraghi AA. **Vitamin A supplementation and serum Th1- and Th2-associated cytokine response in women.** J Am Coll Nutr. 2013;32(4):280-5. doi: 10.1080/07315724.2013.816616. PMID: 24024773.

84 obese and non-obese women were given vitamin A (retinyl palmitate 25,000 IU / d). Conclusions: "Decline in serum concentrations of IL-1β and IL-1β/IL-4 ratio in obese women suggests that vitamin A is capable of regulating the immune system and possibly reducing the risk of autoimmune disease in this group".

Hogarth CA, Griswold MD. **The key role of vitamin A in spermatogenesis.** J Clin Invest. 2010 Apr;120(4):956-62. doi: 10.1172/JCI41303. Epub 2010 Apr 1. PMID: 20364093; PMCID: PMC2846058.

Vitamin A is very important in sperm production and can help with fertilization problems. It is very important for many men, especially because nowadays we have huge problems with fertility. Vitamin A is also essential for the proper development of the fetus.

Ortega RM, Andrés P, Martínez RM, López-Sobaler AM. **Vitamin A status during the third trimester of pregnancy in Spanish women: influence on concentrations of vitamin A in breast milk.** Am J Clin Nutr. 1997 Sep;66(3):564-8. doi: 10.1093/ajcn/66.3.564. PMID: 9280174.

"We conclude from these results that dietary counseling is warranted to ensure adequate vitamin A intake during pregnancy and lactation. Monitoring and improving the vitamin A status of women during this critical period may help improve hepatic stores of vitamin A in children and provide a more adequate amount in breast milk. Both effects may contribute to improvements in nutritional status of young children with respect to vitamin A and this may in turn have a positive effect on their growth and health."

It prevents premature separation of the placenta from the uterine wall and helps the breastfeeding mother to have enough milk.

Basu S, Khanna P, Srivastava R, Kumar A. **Oral vitamin A supplementation in very low birth weight neonates: a randomized controlled trial.** Eur J Pediatr. 2019 Aug;178(8):1255-1265. doi: 10.1007/s00431-019-03412-w. Epub 2019 Jun 17. Erratum in: Eur J Pediatr. 2019 Jul 24;: PMID: 31209560.

Moreover: "Postnatal intramuscular vitamin A supplementation improves the survival, respiratory outcome and other morbidities in very low birth weight neonates without major adverse effects".

It also affects the proper functioning of the thyroid gland.

Farhangi MA, Keshavarz SA, Eshraghian M, Ostadrahimi A, Saboor-Yaraghi AA. **The effect of vitamin A supplementation on thyroid function in premenopausal women.** J Am Coll Nutr. 2012 Aug;31(4):268-74. doi: 10.1080/07315724.2012.10720431. PMID: 23378454.

The research on 84 healthy women aged 17-50 years old showed: "Serum TSH concentrations in vitamin A-treated subjects were significantly reduced; therefore, vitamin A supplementation might reduce the risk of subclinical hypothyroidism in premenopausal women".

High doses of vitamin A (up to 100,000 IU) can help women with heavy menstrual bleeding.

Saboor-Yaraghi AA, Harirchian MH, Mohammadzadeh Honarvar N, Bitarafan S, Abdolahi M, Siassi F, Salehi E, Sahraian MA, Eshraghian MR, Roostaei T, Koohdani F. **The Effect of Vitamin A Supplementation on FoxP3 and TGF-β Gene Expression in Avonex-Treated Multiple Sclerosis Patients.** J Mol Neurosci. 2015 Jul;56(3):608-12. doi: 10.1007/s12031-015-0549-y. Epub 2015 May 19. PMID: 25985851.

Vitamin A can help prevent or treat multiple sclerosis. How many doctors know about that?

itarafan S, Saboor-Yaraghi A, Sahraian MA, Soltani D, Nafissi S, Togha M, Beladi Moghadam N, Roostaei T, Mohammadzadeh Honarvar N, Harirchian MH. **Effect of Vitamin A Supplementation on fatigue and depression in Multiple Sclerosis patients: A Double-Blind Placebo-Controlled Clinical Trial.** Iran J Allergy Asthma Immunol. 2016 Feb;15(1):13-9. PMID: 26996107.

Furthermore, vitamin A has helped with fatigue and depression in patients with multiple sclerosis.

Mottaghi A, Salehi E, Keshvarz A, Sezavar H, Saboor-Yaraghi AA. **The influence of vitamin A supplementation on Foxp3 and TGF-β gene expression in atherosclerotic patients.** J Nutrigenet Nutrigenomics. 2012;5(6):314-26. doi: 10.1159/000341916. Epub 2013 Jan 26. PMID: 23363776.

Mottaghi A, Ebrahimof S, Angoorani P, Saboor-Yaraghi AA. **Vitamin A supplementation reduces IL-17 and RORc gene expression in atherosclerotic patients.** Scand J Immunol. 2014 Aug;80(2):151-7. doi: 10.1111/sji.12190. PMID: 24845870.

Iranian scientists say vitamin A may prove to be helpful in slowing down the progression of atherosclerosis. And aren't the saturated fats of animal origin the richest in vitamin A? Those saturated fats that "cause" atherosclerosis?

People with psoriasis almost always have low vitamin A levels.

To prevent deficiency in a child who is poorly converting beta-carotene, he needs to get his vitamin A from animal sources. Carrot juice may not help here.

Vitamin K2 works together with vitamin A. And

vitamin A is antagonistic to vitamin D. All of these vitamins should be supplemented together.

Johansson S, Melhus H. **Vitamin A antagonizes calcium response to vitamin D in man.** J Bone Miner Res. 2001 Oct;16(10):1899-905. doi: 10.1359/jbmr.2001.16.10.1899. PMID: 11585356.

High intake of this vitamin, with low intake of vitamin D3, can lead to bone problems.

Metz AL, Walser MM, Olson WG. **The interaction of dietary vitamin A and vitamin D related to skeletal development in the turkey poult.** J Nutr. 1985 Jul;115(7):929-35. doi: 10.1093/jn/115.7.929. PMID: 4009300.

"When poults were fed a diet containing high levels of both vitamins A and D growth rate and bone mineral content were similar to control poults fed a diet containing the required levels of vitamins A and D. "

However, when vitamin A and vitamin D were used together, no toxicity occurred regardless of the dose.

Lena Sibulesky, KC Hayes, Andrzej Pronczuk, Carol Weigel-DiFranco, Bernard Rosner, Eliot L Berson, **Safety of <7500 RE (<25000 IU) vitamin A daily in adults with retinitis pigmentosa**, The American Journal of Clinical Nutrition, Volume 69, Issue 4, April 1999, Pages 656–663, https://doi.org/10.1093/ajcn/69.4.656

'Prolonged daily consumption of <7500 RE (<25000 IU) vitamin A/d can be considered safe in this age group".

The use of vitamin A for 2 to 12 years showed no liver damage or other harmful effects.

The first symptoms of vitamin A poisoning may appear after supplementing with 100,000 IU a day for six months or more. Several studies have also concluded that synthetically produced beta-carotene may promote cancer development. This does not apply to natural beta-carotene.

High vitamin A foods per 100g:
- Lamb Liver Cooked - 7782µg (865% DV)
- Pan Fried Beef Liver - 7744µg (860% DV)
- King Mackerel - 252µg (28% DV)
- Salmon - 149µg (17% DV)
- Cheddar - 330µg (37% DV)
- Butter - 684µg (76% DV)
- Hard-Boiled Egg - 149µg (17% DV)

VITAMIN E

Vitamin E is two main groups of substances: tocopherols and tocotrienols
Each of them consists of four subgroups:

- alpha tocopherol, beta tocopherol, delta tocopherol, gamma tocopherol
- alpha tocotrienol, beta tocotrienol, delta tocotrienol, gamma tocotrienol

Alpha, gamma and delta tocopherol together exhibit antioxidant activity. Interestingly, tocotrienols are 40 to 60 times more potent antioxidants than alpha tocopherol. It's a big misunderstanding when someone talks about vitamin E in general and says it doesn't work. Either he has a financial interest in not saying all, or he just doesn't know anything about vitamin E.

Kooyenga DK, Geller M, Watkins TR, Gapor A, Diakoumakis E, Bierenbaum ML. **Palm oil antioxidant effects in patients with hyperlipidaemia and carotid stenosis-2 year experience.** Asia Pac J Clin Nutr. 1997 Mar;6(1):72-5. PMID: 24394659.

Scientists have shown that a mixture of tocotrienols from palm seeds allowed to remove cholesterol deposits from the arteries in about 6 months.

Theriault A, Chao JT, Gapor A. **Tocotrienol is the most effective vitamin E for reducing endothelial expression of adhesion molecules and adhesion to monocytes. Atherosclerosis.** 2002 Jan;160(1):21-30. doi: 10.1016/s0021-9150(01)00540-8. Erratum in: Atherosclerosis. 2002;164(2):389.. Chao, Jun Tzu [corrected to Chao, Jun-Tzu]; Gapor, Abeli [corrected to Gapor, Abdul]. PMID: 11755919.

Chao JT, Gapor A, Theriault A. **Inhibitory effect of delta-tocotrienol, a HMG CoA reductase inhibitor, on monocyte-endothelial cell adhesion.** J Nutr Sci Vitaminol (Tokyo). 2002 Oct;48(5):332-7. doi: 10.3177/jnsv.48.332. PMID: 12656204.

Delta tocotrienol, in particular, may support arterial health and prove useful in treating.

Newaz MA, Yousefipour Z, Nawal N, Adeeb N. **Nitric oxide synthase activity in blood vessels of spontaneously hypertensive rats: antioxidant protection by gamma-tocotrienol.** J Physiol Pharmacol. 2003

Sep;54(3):319-27. PMID: 14566071.

This vitamin can help regulate blood pressure.

Theriault A, Chao JT, Wang Q, Gapor A, Adeli K. **Tocotrienol: a review of its therapeutic potential**. Clin Biochem. 1999 Jul;32(5):309-19. doi: 10.1016/s0009-9120(99)00027-2. PMID: 10480444.

"Interestingly, tocotrienols have been shown to reduce plasma cholesterol levels, as well as, other lipid and non-lipid related risk factors for CVD"
Lowering the level of LDL cholesterol and triglycerides occurs with supplementation with tocotrienols in amounts ranging from 100 mg to 200 mg per day.

Wong WY, Ward LC, Fong CW, Yap WN, Brown L. **Anti-inflammatory γ- and δ-tocotrienols improve cardiovascular, liver and metabolic function in diet-induced obese rats.** Eur J Nutr. 2017 Feb;56(1):133-150. doi: 10.1007/s00394-015-1064-1. Epub 2015 Oct 8. PMID: 26446095.

"In rats, δ-tocotrienol improved inflammation, heart structure and function, and liver structure and function, while γ-tocotrienol produced more modest improvements, with minimal changes with α-tocotrienol and α-tocopherol. The most important mechanism of action is likely to be reduction in organ inflammation".

This may be related to the anti-inflammatory effects of tocotrienols.

Theriault A, Chao JT, Wang Q, Gapor A, Adeli K. **Tocotrienol: a review of its therapeutic potential.** Clin Biochem. 1999 Jul;32(5):309-19. doi: 10.1016/s0009-9120(99)00027-2. PMID: 10480444.

Tocotrienols in particular can prevent or have a positive effect on diseases of the nervous system.

Ismail M, Alsalahi A, Imam MU, Ooi J, Khaza'ai H, Aljaberi MA, Shamsudin MN, Idrus Z. **Safety and Neuroprotective Efficacy of Palm Oil and Tocotrienol-Rich Fraction from Palm Oil:** A Systematic Review. Nutrients. 2020 Feb 18;12(2):521. doi: 10.3390/nu12020521. PMID: 32085610; PMCID: PMC7071496.

In this publication from 2020, the researchers concluded that Palm oil and its tocotrienol-rich fraction enhanced the cognitive functions of healthy animals. It is also related to attenuation of oxidative stress.

I must also mention the remarkable role of vitamin E in preventing and treating cancer. Why is nobody talking about it despite the multitude of scientific publications on the subject? Here are a few of them:

McAnally JA, Gupta J, Sodhani S, Bravo L, Mo H. **Tocotrienols potentiate lovastatin-mediated growth suppression in vitro and in vivo.** Exp Biol Med (Maywood). 2007 Apr;232(4):523-31. PMID: 17392488.

Mo, Huanbiao & Elfakhani, Manal & Shah, Anureet & Yeganehjoo, Hoda. (2012). **Mevalonate-Suppressive Tocotrienols for Cancer Chemoprevention and Adjuvant Therapy.** 10.1201/b12502-11.

Nesaretnam K, Stephen R, Dils R, Darbre P. **Tocotrienols inhibit the growth of human breast cancer cells irrespective of estrogen receptor status.** Lipids. 1998 May;33(5):461-9. doi: 10.1007/s11745-998-0229-3. PMID: 9625593.

Conte C, Floridi A, Aisa C, Piroddi M, Floridi A, Galli F. **Gamma-tocotrienol metabolism and antiproliferative effect in prostate cancer cells.** Ann N Y Acad Sci. 2004 Dec;1031:391-4. doi: 10.1196/annals.1331.054. PMID: 15753178.

Idriss M, Hodroj MH, Fakhoury R, Rizk S. **Beta-Tocotrienol Exhibits More Cytotoxic Effects than Gamma-Tocotrienol on Breast Cancer Cells by Promoting Apoptosis via a P53-Independent PI3-Kinase Dependent Pathway.** Biomolecules. 2020 Apr 9;10(4):577. doi: 10.3390/biom10040577. PMID: 32283796; PMCID: PMC7226046.

"These findings suggest that vitamin E beta-T3 should be considered as a promising anti-cancer agent, more effective than gamma-T3 for treating human breast cancer and deserves to be further studied to investigate its effects in vitro and on other cancer types."

Fontana F, Moretti RM, Raimondi M, Marzagalli M, Beretta G, Procacci P, Sartori P, Montagnani Marelli M, Limonta P. **δ-Tocotrienol induces apoptosis, involving endoplasmic reticulum stress and autophagy, and paraptosis in prostate cancer cells.** Cell Prolif. 2019 May;52(3):e12576. doi: 10.1111/cpr.12576. Epub 2019 Feb 4. PMID: 30719778; PMCID: PMC6536411.

Only tocotrienols can help prevent and slow the growth of cancer cells in the liver, prostate, breast, lung, colon and pancreas. Delta tocotrienol is the most effective component of vitamin E and, in addition to inhibiting the growth of cancer cells, it induces the process of apoptosis (It is a natural process of programmed and controlled cell destruction). Isn't it extremely important for those who want to prevent cancer and those who are already fighting it? Why has nobody taken any action on the facts above? We can guess the answer...

Mizushina Y, Nakagawa K, Shibata A, Awata Y, Kuriyama I, Shimazaki N, Koiwai O, Uchiyama Y, Sakaguchi K, Miyazawa T, Yoshida H. **Inhibitory effect of tocotrienol on eukaryotic DNA polymerase lambda and angiogenesis.** Biochem Biophys Res Commun. 2006 Jan 20;339(3):949-55. doi: 10.1016/j.bbrc.2005.1-1.085. Epub 2005 Nov 28. PMID: 16325764.

Tocotrienols also inhibit the growth of new blood vessels in the tumor.

For better effectiveness, during the supplementation, tocopherols and tocotrienols should be taken separately.

McIntyre BS, Briski KP, Tirmenstein MA, Fariss MW, Gapor A, Sylvester PW. **Antiproliferative and apoptotic effects of tocopherols and tocotrienols on normal mouse mammary epithelial cells.** Lipids. 2000 Feb;35(2):171-80. doi: 10.1007/BF0266-4767. PMID: 10757548.

"Results also showed that mammary epithelial cells more easily or preferentially took up tocotrienols as compared to tocopherols, suggesting that at least part of the reason tocotrienols display greater biopotency than tocopherols is because of greater cellular accumulation."

u SG, Thomas AM, Gapor A, Tan B, Qureshi N, Qureshi AA. **Dose-response impact of various tocotrienols on serum lipid parameters in 5-week-old female chickens.** Lipids. 2006 May;41(5):453-61. doi: 10.1007/s11745-006-5119-1. PMID: 16933790.

The most commonly sold form of vitamin E, i. e. alpha tocopherol, shows almost no effectiveness. It is not worth wasting money on this form. Delta tocotrienol shows the highest effectiveness. In second place is gamma tocotrienol.

High vitamin E foods in milligrams per 100g:
- Sunflower oil - 65
- Palm oil - 33
- Sunflower seeds - 35
- Almonds - 24
- Rapeseed oil - 23
- Olive oil - 13

VITAMIN C

There is also a lot of misunderstanding in the world about vitamin C. Determining the need for vitamin C is not easy and straightforward. The same recommendations for everyone are absurd. Vitamin C half-life varies from 8 to 40 days when blood levels of vitamin C are low. In this way, the body protects itself against scurvy. When our blood levels of vitamin C are high then the half-life is only 30 minutes. Experienced Dr. Robert F. Cathcart, who treated with high doses of vitamin C, noticed that the body significantly increases the consumption of vitamin C during inflammation, surgery, bacterial infections and emotional stress. In such cases, vitamin C can even drop to almost zero. A bee sting or a small infection can drastically change the vitamin C levels (which hardly anyone knows).

Cathcart RF. **Vitamin C, titrating to bowel tolerance, anascorbemia, and acute induced scurvy.** Med Hypotheses. 1981 Nov;7(11):1359-76. doi: 10.1016/0306-9877(81)90126-2. PMID: 7321921.

The same doctor noted that the amount of orally

administered vitamin C that can be tolerated by the digestive system without causing diarrhea is more than 10 times greater in a sick organism than when the same person is healthy. The "subthreshold" amount of vitamin C is considered by practitioners to be the most effective. We check the tolerance subthreshold by gradually giving vitamin C every hour or two until mild diarrhea occurs. When mild diarrhea occurs, we reduce the amount of vitamin C a little and still continue. This way, you can get rid of many infections very quickly.

Ausman LM. **Criteria and recommendations for vitamin C intake**. Nutr Rev. 1999 Jul;57(7):222-4. doi: 10.1111/j.1753-4887.1999.tb06946.x. PMID: 10453176.

High doses of vitamin C are not toxic.
Dr Cathcart gives what amounts and in what doses he administered vitamin C for a particular disease:
- *cold: 30-60 grams daily in 6-10 doses.*
- *severe cold: 60-100+ grams daily in 8-15 doses.*
- *flu: 100-150 grams daly in 8-20 doses.*
- *asthma, hay fever: 15-50 grams daily in 4-8 doses.*
- *viral pneumonia: 100-200+ grams daily in 12-25 doses.*
- *allergy: 0,5-50 grams daily in 4-8 doses.*
- *rheumatoid arthritis: 15-100 grams daily in 4-15*

doses.

- bacterial infections: 30-200+ grams daily in 10-25 doses.

- candidiasis: 15-200+ grams daily in 6-25 doses.

Cathcart RF 3rd. **Vitamin C: the nontoxic, non-rate-limited, antioxidant free radical scavenger.** Med Hypotheses. 1985 Sep;18(1):61-77. doi: 10.1016/0306-9877(85)90121-5. PMID: 4069036.

Sodium ascorbate is better tolerated than ascorbic acid in high doses. For intravenous infusions, sodium ascorbate is always and only used. Intravenous infusions should be done by a person who has experience and extensive knowledge in this subject.

Here I recommend to read the RECNAC project on which Neil H. Riordan, Hugh D. Riordan and Ronald E. Hunninghake worked on. They discussed the topic of intravenous infusions very thoroughly.

I also recommend for those more interested in the topic:

Challem, J., Gonzalez, M., Levy, T., Hunninghake, R., & Matalon, V. (2009). Roundtable: **Intravenous Vitamin C for Treating Cancer. Alternative and Complementary Therapies**, 15 (2), 81-86.

Clinical Guide to the Use of Vitamin C. **The Clinical Experiences of Frederick R. Klenner, M. D.** abbreviated, summarized and annotated by Lendon H. Smith, M. D.

Hemilä H. **Vitamin C supplementation and respiratory infections**: a systematic review. Mil Med. 2004 Nov;169(11):920-5. doi: 10.7205/ milmed.169.11.920. PMID: 15605943.

Vitamin C increases the activity of white blood cells and reduces viral replication. The degree of pathogen neutralization in a viral infection is proportional to the concentration of vitamin C and, very importantly, the length of time it is administered. The symptoms of chickenpox and mumps can also be significantly reduced in the short term following vitamin C administration. Could people with Covid-19 also be treated with effective, safe and cheap vitamin C? The answer is obvious and medical practice has already confirmed it. Moreover, if we began to maintain proper vitamin D levels (as I have already mentioned) in society and use vitamin C (mainly intravenous infusions), zinc, selenium, vitamin E and iodine in hospitals, we could end the Covid-19 pandemic in about two weeks.

"Vitamin C helps control virus infections, and if

there is a failure, usually it is because not enough C was being used."

Dr. Klenner concluded: "The degree of neutralization in a virus infection will be in proportion to the concentration of the vitamin and the length of time which it is employed". The lack of the terephthalic effect of vitamin C is usually associated with too little vitamin C and too short a period of its use.

Vitamin C can be of great importance in the prevention and treatment of cancer.

Ewan Cameron and Linus Pauling found that when a cancer patient (classified as incurable) was given only 10 g / day of vitamin C, these patients survived an average of 300 days longer than those in the control group. 22% of patients survived for more than one year compared to 0.4% in the control group.

Cameron E, Pauling L. **Supplemental ascorbate in the supportive treatment of cancer: reevaluation of prolongation of survival times in terminal human cancer.** Proc Natl Acad Sci U S A. 1978 Sep;75(9):4538-42. doi: 10.1073/pnas.75.9.4538. PMID: 279931; PMCID: PMC336151.

The results of the retry turned out to be even better.

Hong SW, Jin DH, Hahm ES, Yim SH, Lim JS, Kim KI, Yang Y, Lee SS, Kang JS, Lee WJ, Lee WK, Lee MS. **Ascorbate (vitamin C) induces cell death through the apoptosis-inducing factor in human breast cancer cells.** Oncol Rep. 2007 Oct;18(4):811-5. PMID: 17786340.

The above studies show that vitamin C destroys breast cancer cells by causing natural cell death (apoptosis).

Lee SK, Kang JS, Jung DJ, Hur DY, Kim JE, Hahm E, Bae S, Kim HW, Kim D, Cho BJ, Cho D, Shin DH, Hwang YI, Lee WJ. **Vitamin C suppresses proliferation of the human melanoma cell SK-MEL-2 through the inhibition of cyclooxygenase-2 (COX-2) expression and the modulation of insulin-like growth factor II (IGF-II) production.** J Cell Physiol. 2008 Jul;216(1):180-8. doi: 10.1002/jcp.21391. PMID: 18297687.

Korean scientists have shown that vitamin C inhibits the growth of skin cancer cells.

Uetaki, M., Tabata, S., Nakasuka, F. et al. **Metabolomic alterations in human cancer cells by vitamin C-induced oxidative stress.** Sci Rep 5, 13896

(2015). https://doi.org/10.1038/sre-p13896

Vitamin C contributes to the induction of apoptosis in various types of neoplastic cells, e. g. pancreas and leukemia.

Hardin Jones Biostatistical Analysis of **Mortality Data for Cohorts of Cancer Patients with a Large Fraction Surviving at the Termination of the Study and a Comparison of Survival Times of Cancer Patients Receiving Large Regular Oral Doses of Vitamin C and Other Nutrients with Similar Patients Not Receiving Those Doses** A. Hoffer, M. D., Ph. D. and Linus Pauling, Ph. D. 1990

In a study of 134 cancer patients with an average age of 53.1 years, two groups received an average of 12 g / day of vitamin C and a third group was a control group that was not receiving vitamin C. They found that 80% of the patients who took vitamin C had a life expectancy of 21 times greater than that of the control group.

Hardin Jones Biostatistical Analysis of **Mortality Data for a Second Set of Cohorts of Cancer Patients with a Large Fraction Surviving at the Termination of the Study and a Comparison of Survival Times of Cancer Patients Receiving Large Regular Oral Doses of Vitamin C and Other Nutrients with**

Similar Patients Not Receiving These Doses

A. Hoffer, M. D., Ph. D. and Linus Pauling, Ph. D. 1993

The results of studies by the same authors, with treatment with also other nutrients:

"In the extended first study about 50% of the patients with cancer of the breast and related organs are estimated to be excellent responders, with mean survival time greater than 5 years (1827 days), with the other 50% being good responders, with mean survival time 630 days. For the patients with other kinds of cancer it is estimated that about 33% are excellent responders, with mean survival time greater than 5 years, and 67% are good responders, with mean survival time 540 days (...) The good responders have mean survival time about 4 times that of the controls. "

Waring AJ, Drake IM, Schorah CJ, et al. **Ascorbic acid and total vitamin C concentrations in plasma, gastric juice, and gastrointestinal mucosa: effects of gastritis and oral supplementation.** Gut. 1996;38(2):171-176. doi:10.1136/gut.38.2.171

High vitamin C content in the diet also reduces the risk of stomach cancer.

Carr AC, Vissers MC, Cook JS. **The effect of intravenous vitamin C on cancer- and chemotherapy-related fatigue and quality of life**. Front Oncol. 2014;4:283. Published 2014 Oct 16. doi:10.3389/fonc.2014.00283

Intravenous vitamin C relieves a number of symptoms related to cancer and chemotherapy, such as pain, fatigue, insomnia, loss of appetite, and nausea.

Błasiak J, Gloc E, Woźniak K, Młynarski W, Stolarska M, Skórski T, Majsterek I. **Genotoxicity of idarubicin and its modulation by vitamins C and E and amifostine**. Chem Biol Interact. 2002 Apr 20;140(1):1-18. doi: 10.1016/s0009-2797(02)00012-1. PMID: 12044557.

"Vitamin C can be considered as protective agents against DNA damage in normal cells in persons receiving idarubicin-based chemotherapy (...)"
It can therefore reduce the side effects of chemotherapy. Few know about the above-mentioned effect of vitamin C. Shouldn't we talk more about it, especially since we have a cancer epidemic all over the world? While academic medicine cannot cope with cancer almost in general, the number of cancers is increasing.

Vitamin C can save lives in another case as well...

Wilson JX. **Mechanism of action of vitamin C in sepsis: ascorbate modulates redox signaling in endothelium**. Biofactors. 2009;35(1):5-13. doi:10.1002/biof.7

Wilson JX. **Evaluation of vitamin C for adjuvant sepsis therapy**. Antioxid Redox Signal. 2013;19(17):2129-2140. doi:10.1089/ars.2013.5401

Carr AC, Shaw GM, Fowler AA, Natarajan R. **Ascorbate-dependent vasopressor synthesis: a rationale for vitamin C administration in severe sepsis and septic shock?** Crit Care. 2015;19:418. Published 2015 Nov 27. doi:10.1186/s13054-015-1131-2

Sepsis, the state of the body in which a huge amount of free radicals has been formed as a result of the action of bacteria or viruses, can be overcome by vitamin C.

Mikirova, Nina & Rogers, AM & Casciari, Joseph & Taylor, Paul. (2012). **Effect of high dose intravenous ascorbic acid on the level of inflammation in patients with rheumatoid arthritis.** Modern Research in Inflammation. 01. 26-32. 10.4236/mri. 2012.12004.

Vitamin C given intravenously can greatly help with rheumatoid arthritis:
"Our data suggest that IVC therapy with dosages of 7.5 g-50 g can reduce inflammation. The level of inflammation as measured by C-reactive protein levels was decreased on average by 44%. Based on our pilot study, we hypothesize that IVC therapy can be a useful strategy in treating RA."

Oudemans-van Straaten HM, Spoelstra-de Man AM, de Waard MC. **Vitamin C revisited**. Crit Care. 2014 Aug 6;18(4):460. doi: 10.1186/s13054-014-0460-x. PMID: 25185110; PMCID: PMC4423646.

Vitamin C has a positive effect on the circulatory system and, in an appropriately high dose, can prevent vessel damage by reactive oxygen species.

Aguirre R, May JM. **Inflammation in the vascular bed: importance of vitamin C**. Pharmacol Ther. 2008;119(1):96-103. doi:10.1016/j.pharmthera.2008.05.002

"Although further studies of ascorbate function in these cell types and in novel animal models are needed, available evidence generally supports a salutary role for this vitamin in ameliorating the earliest stages of atherosclerosis."

It can also help reverse the early stages of atherosclerosis. Vitamin C deficiency can increase the risk of developing atherosclerotic plaque and increase the risk of stroke. This can be due to impaired collagen synthesis and reduced NOS (Nitric oxide synthases) production. Vitamin C works here on two levels. First, it neutralizes free radicals that destroy the endothelium. Secondly, it supports the proper structure of collagen.

Hansen SN, Tveden-Nyborg P, Lykkesfeldt J. **Does vitamin C deficiency affect cognitive development and function?** Nutrients. 2014 Sep 19;6(9):3818-46. doi: 10.3390/nu6093818. PMID: 25244370; PMCID: PMC4179190.

In addition, vitamin C lowers blood pressure in patients with mild to moderately high blood pressure. Vitamin C affects the proper functioning of the brain and well-being.

Hansen SN, Tveden-Nyborg P, Lykkesfeldt J. **Does vitamin C deficiency affect cognitive development and function?** Nutrients. 2014 Sep 19;6(9):3818-46. doi: 10.3390/nu6093818. PMID: 25244370; PMCID: PMC4179190.

It modulates the brain's neurotransmitter system. Vitamin C contributes to the development of new blood vessels (angiogenesis) and participates in the maturation of neurons and the formation of myelin. It is also involved in transmitting signals through the nervous system by neurotransmitters.

Brody S. **High-dose ascorbic acid increases intercourse frequency and improves mood**: a randomized controlled clinical trial. Biol Psychiatry. 2002 Aug 15;52(4):371-4. doi: 10.1016/s0006-3223(02)01329-x. PMID: 12208645.

Vitamin C increases the release of oxytocin. Furthermore, vitamin C deficiencies are associated with nervousness and emotional instability.

de Oliveira IJ, de Souza VV, Motta V, Da-Silva SL. **Effects of Oral Vitamin C Supplementation on Anxiety in Students**: A Double-Blind, Randomized, Placebo-Controlled Trial. Pak J Biol Sci. 2015 Jan;18(1):11-8. doi: 10.3923/pjbs.2015.11.18. PMID: 26353411.

"Present study results not only provide evidence that vitamin C plays an important therapeutic role for anxiety but also point a possible use for antioxidants in the prevention or reduction of anxiety. This suggests that a diet rich in vitamin C may be an effective adjunct to medical and psychological treatment of anxiety and improve academic performance."

Taking vitamin C reduced anxiety in high school students.

Vitamin C can help treat depression

Johnston CS, Barkyoumb GM, Schumacher SS. **Vitamin C supplementation slightly improves physical activity levels and reduces cold incidence in men with marginal vitamin C status**: a randomized controlled trial. Nutrients. 2014;6(7):2572-2583. Published 2014 Jul 9. doi:10.3390/nu6072572

Vitamin C is necessary for the conversion of neurotransmitters - hormones which transformation is disturbed during depression, and if the level of vitamin C is too low, symptoms of depression worsen. Vitamin C may also increase the effectiveness of antidepressants.

Amr M, El-Mogy A, Shams T, Vieira K, Lakhan SE. **Efficacy of vitamin C as an adjunct to fluoxetine therapy in pediatric major depressive disorder:** a randomized, double-blind, placebo-controlled pilot study. Nutr J. 2013 Mar 9;12:31.

doi: 10.1186/1475-2891-12-31. PMID: 23510529; PMCID: PMC3599706.

"These results show that orally administered vitamin C as an adjunct to fluoxetine treatment leads to significantly greater decreases in depressive symptoms in comparison to fluoxetine treatment alone." Vitamin C improves the mood of healthy people and reduces the severity of depressive disorders in children and adults.

Hansen SN, Tveden-Nyborg P, Lykkesfeldt J. **Does vitamin C deficiency affect cognitive development and function?** Nutrients. 2014 Sep 19;6(9):3818-46. doi: 10.3390/nu6093818. PMID: 25244370; PMCID: PMC4179190.

Chronic vitamin C deficiency affects the formation and development of neurodegenerative disorders, and vitamin C supplementation may reduce the risk of Alzheimer's disease.

Harrison FE. **A critical review of vitamin C for the prevention of age-related cognitive decline and Alzheimer's disease.** J Alzheimers Dis. 2012;29(4):711-726. doi:10.3233/JAD-2012-111853

Furthermore, increasing vitamin C intake may improve cognition in the elderly.

Vitamin C plays a very important role in the production of collagen. Therefore, it affects the proper structure of the connective tissue of the skin, bones, cartilage, tendons, ligaments and blood vessels.

Vitamin C helps in detoxification of heavy metals. About 5 grams of vitamin C removes: 20.7 µg of lead, 20.0 µg of mercury, 7.5 µg of arsenic, 11.2 µg of cadmium and 5.6 µg of nickel.

Nakhostin-Roohi B, Babaei P, Rahmani-Nia F, Bohlooli S. **Effect of vitamin C supplementation on lipid peroxidation, muscle damage and inflammation after 30-min exercise at 75% VO2max**. J Sports Med Phys Fitness. 2008 Jun;48(2):217-24. PMID: 18427418.

Vitamin C may also prove useful during exercise due to the reduction of oxidative stress and thus prevent, for example, muscle damage.

Vitamin C may be necessary after and before surgery when the body is weakened and the amount of vitamin C is very low.

In the case of severe burns, including sunburn or

sunstroke, vitamin C administered intravenously can greatly improve the health situation. And: "One gram taken every one to two hours during exposure will prevent sunburn".

Due to the specificity of vitamin C, it helps, to a greater or lesser extent, with almost all ailments.

Curhan GC, Willett WC, Speizer FE, Stampfer MJ. **Intake of vitamins B6 and C and the risk of kidney stones in women.** J Am Soc Nephrol. 1999 Apr;10(4):840-5. PMID: 10203369.

Schmidt KH, Hagmaier V, Hornig DH, Vuilleumier JP, Rutishauser G. **Urinary oxalate excretion after large intakes of ascorbic acid in man.** Am J Clin Nutr. 1981 Mar;34(3):305-11. doi: 10.1093/ajcn/34.3.305. PMID: 7211731.

Wandzilak TR, D'Andre SD, Davis PA, Williams HE. **Effect of high dose vitamin C on urinary oxalate levels.** J Urol. 1994 Apr;151(4):834-7. doi: 10.1016/s0022-5347(17)35100-5. PMID: 8126804.

Gerster H. **No contribution of ascorbic acid to renal calcium oxalate stones.** Ann Nutr Metab. 1997;41(5):269-82. doi: 10.1159/000177954. PMID: 9429689.

Vitamin C does not cause kidney stones. It has been proven many times and such nonsense is still repeated in universities. People with kidney disease, haemochromatosis and von Gierke disease should consult a specialist in the case of using higher doses of vitamin C. Diarrhea is the most common side effect.

More than 4,000 species of mammals produce vitamin C. The production of vitamin C by these animals per kg of body weight compared to human weight would not be in milligrams but grams. For example, goats produce huge 200 mg / kg of vitamin C daily, while for humans, around 1 mg of vitamin C per kilogram of body weight is recommended. For health, Dr. Levy recommends 6-9 grams of ascorbic acid or 2 grams of liposomal vitamin C (which is effective on a daily basis and in treatment, but administered in a smaller amount. 1 gram of liposomal vitamin C equals about 10 grams of ascorbic acid). Linus Pauling recommended 6-18 grams per day.

VITAMIN B1 (THIAMIN)

Thiamin participates in the metabolism of amino acids and carbohydrates as a coenzyme for enzymes.

Lonsdale D. **A review of the biochemistry, metabolism and clinical benefits of thiamin (e) and its derivatives**. Evid Based Complement Alternat Med. 2006 Mar;3(1):49-59. doi: 10.1093/ecam/nek009. PMID: 16550223; PMCID: PMC1375232.

The body needs thiamine to make adenosine triphosphate (ATP). This is a molecule that transports energy within cells. It helps also in converting carbohydrates into glucose as well as metabolizing proteins and fats. Therefore, among other things, people with diabetes should remember about this vitamin.

Thinking and remembering improve after vitamin B1 supplementation. A deficiency of this vitamin causes nervousness, anger attacks, learning difficulties and depression. The administration of 50 mg of vitamin B1 in people with normal levels improves their mood and brain function. It is also called the mood vitamin by some. Thiamin contributes to the improved functioning of the nervous system and supports the cardiovascular system. For example, Vitamin B1 helps to form the myelin sheath that protects the nerves from damage in rats with a deficiency of thiamine.

Costantini A, Pala MI, Catalano ML, Notarangelo C, Careddu P. **High-dose thiamine improves fatigue after stroke: a report of three cases.** J Altern Complement Med. 2014 Sep;20(9):683-5. doi: 10.1089/acm.2013.0461. PMID: 25192035.

High doses of thiamine have also been shown to reduce fatigue in stroke patients.

Thiamine has also a beneficial effect on neurodegenerative diseases such as Parkinson's disease, Alzheimer's disease, Wernicke's encephalopathy, and Huntington's disease.

Pletsityi, A.D. **Changes in activity of some mechanisms of specific and nonspecific immunity in vitamin B1 deficiency.** Bull Exp Biol Med 88, 741–743 (1979). https://doi.org/10.1007/B-F00804782

It is believed to improve the proper functioning of the immune system. Also, find out that thiamin has antioxidant results. Vitamin B1 is essential for enzymes to protect cells and mitochondria from oxidative stress. Its deficiency can damage cells in the central nervous system. Oxidative stress can also be caused by changes in carbohydrate metabolism.

Researchers at Warwick University (UK) have shown that adequate vitamin B1 doses can reverse early kidney damage in people with type 2 diabetes. Studies have shown that the loss of protein in the urine (which is a symptom of kidney damage) decreased under the influence of a high dose of vitamin B1 administered for 3 months.

Earlier studies by the same researchers showed that 70-90 percent of people struggling with type 1 and type 2 diabetes are deficient in vitamin B1. They have also looked at thiamine as a possible treatment for kidney disease and cataracts.

Vitamin B1 is also necessary for the functioning of the digestive system. It helps to regulate the production of hydrochloric acid.

People who are undergoing dialysis for their kidneys or taking loop diuretics are at risk for thiamine deficiency.

Ideally, vitamin B1 should be administered with magnesium, vitamin B6 and zinc.

High vitamin B1 foods per 100g:
- Lean Pork Chop (56% DV)
- Fish - Salmon (28% DV) and in a 6oz tuna fillet (39% DV)
- Flax Seeds (137% DV) and in 1oz of sunflower seeds (36% DV)
- Navy Beans (20% DV) and in 1 cup of black beans (35% DV)
- Green Peas (22% DV) and asparagus (14% DV)

VITAMIN B2 (RIBOFLAVIN)

Vitamin B2 is an essential component for energy production in the mitochondria.

Vitamin B2 participates in the transport of oxygen in the eye lens and thus protects against cataracts. Riboflavin supplementation inhibits the clouding of the eye lens.

Moat SJ, Ashfield-Watt PA, Powers HJ, Newcombe RG, McDowell IF. **Effect of riboflavin status on the homocysteine-lowering effect of folate in relation to the MTHFR (C677T) genotype.** Clin Chem. 2003 Feb;49(2):295-302. doi: 10.1373/49.2.295. PMID: 12560354.

Vitamin B2 helps maintain the circulatory system in good condition. Riboflavin and folic acid taken together are effective in lowering homocysteine levels.

Horigan G, McNulty H, Ward M, Strain JJ, Purvis J, Scott JM. **Riboflavin lowers blood pressu-**

re in cardiovascular disease patients homozygo-us for the 677C--> T polymorphism in MTHFR. J Hypertens. 2010 Mar;28(3):478-86. doi: 10.1097/HJH.0b013e328334c126. PMID: 19952781.

In people with cardiovascular disease (specifically in patients with the MTHFR 677 TT genotype.), ri-boflavin is effective in lowering blood pressure.

It enhances the effect of insulin. Vitamin B2 is also necessary for the secretion of cortisol. It takes part in the processes of oxidation and reduction, as well as in the transformation of amino acids and lipids. Together with vitamin A, riboflavin affects the mucous membranes, respiratory tract, gastrointe-stinal mucosa, blood vessel epithelium and skin. It is also suspected that riboflavin is involved in the formation of red blood cells and blood. Performs re-gulatory functions important for the entire body.

Siassi F, Ghadirian P. **Riboflavin deficiency and esophageal cancer: a case control-household stu-dy in the Caspian Littoral of Iran**. Can-cer Detect Prev. 2005;29(5):464-9. doi: 10.1016/j.cdp.2005.08.001. Epub 2005 Sep 23. PMID: 16183212.

Vitamin B2 can prevent cancer. Taking vitamin B2 lowered the risk of developing colorectal cancer in women.

It ensures the proper functioning of the nervous system.

Namazi N, Heshmati J, Tarighat-Esfanjani A. **Supplementation with Riboflavin (Vitamin B2) for Migraine Prophylaxis in Adults and Children**: A Review. Int J Vitam Nutr Res. 2015;85(1-2):79-87. doi: 10.1024/0300-9831/a000225. PMID: 26780280.

Vitamin B2 may help prevent migraine headache. Adequately high doses of vitamin B2 prevent the symptoms of migraine. Vitamin B2 supplementation may play a positive role in reducing the frequency and duration of migraine attacks without side effects.

Gaul C, Diener HC, Danesch U; Migravent® Study Group. **Improvement of migraine symptoms with a proprietary supplement containing riboflavin, magnesium and Q10**: a randomized, placebo-controlled, double-blind, multicenter trial. J Headache Pain. 2015;16:516. doi:10.1186/s10194-015-0516-6

Vitamin B2 in combination with magnesium and

coenzyme Q10 can bring even better results.

Vitamin B2 helps prevent cognitive decline. Higher dietary intake of riboflavin is associated with improved cognitive functions in the elderly.

Bell IR, Edman JS, Morrow FD, Marby DW, Perrone G, Kayne HL Greenwald M, Cole JO. Brief communication. **Vitamin B1, B2, and B6 augmentation of tricyclic antidepressant treatment in geriatric depression with cognitive dysfunction.** J Am Coll Nutr. 1992 Apr;11(2):159-63. PMID: 1578091.

People with depression are deficient in riboflavin. Supplementation of B vitamins (including B1, B2, B6) in elderly people with depression improved their well-being.

The increased demand for this vitamin occurs during the period of intensive growth, pregnancy, lactation, and during intense physical exertion and stress.

According to Oregon State University, the recommended daily allowance (RDA) of vitamin B2 for men aged 19 years and over is 1.3 milligrams per day, and for women, it is 1.1 milligram per day.
High vitamin B2 foods per 100g:

- Beef liver (201% DV)
- Beef - Skirt Steak (66% DV)
- Fortified Tofu (34% DV)
- Salmon (37% DV)
- Mushrooms and 1 cup of portabella mushrooms (38% DV)
- Lean Pork Chops (21% DV) and in 1 cup of lean roast ham (36% DV)
- Spinach (18% DV) and 32% DV in 1 cup of beet greens
- Almonds (88% DV)
- Avocados (10% DV)
- Eggs (39% DV)

Vitamin B2 is water soluble, so cooking foods can cause it to be lost.

VITAMIN B3 (NIACIN)

Niacin is essential for the proper functioning of the brain and peripheral nervous system.

Goel H, Dunbar RL. **Niacin Alternatives for Dyslipidemia: Fool's Gold or Gold Mine? Part II: Novel Niacin Mimetics**. Curr Atheroscler Rep. 2016 Apr;18(4):17. doi: 10.1007/s11883-016-0570-9. PMID: 26932224; PMCID: PMC4773474.

The daily intake of an adequate amount of vitamin B3 prevents coronary heart disease and heart failure.

ALTSCHUL R, HOFFER A, STEPHEN JD. **Influence of nicotinic acid on serum cholesterol in man**. Arch Biochem Biophys. 1955 Feb;54(2):558-9. doi: 10.1016/0003-9861(55)90070-9. PMID: 14350806.

Niacin has been used since the 1950 s to treat high cholesterol. However, studies show that niacin raises HDL levels by 15–35% and can also lower triglycerides by 20–50%. Who except the readers of this book knows about it? Few. And heart disease is the number one death factor in the US.

McKenney J. **New Perspectives on the Use of Niacin in the Treatment of Lipid Disorders.** Arch Intern Med. 2004;164(7):6-97–705. doi:10.1001/archinte.164.7.697

Nasser Figueiredo V, Vendrame F, Colontoni BA, Quinaglia T, Roberto Matos-Souza J, Azevedo Moura F, Coelho OR, de Faria EC, Sposito AC. **Short-term effects of extended-release niacin with and without the addition of laropiprant on endothelial function in individuals with low HDL-C: a randomized, controlled crossover trial.** Clin Ther. 2014 Jun 1;36(6):961-6. doi: 10.1016/j.clinthera.2014.03.012. Epub 2014 Apr 24. PMID: 24768191.

Niacin lowers levels of triglycerides and total cholesterol. It also reduces the amount of lipoprotein and limits the accumulation of lipids in the liver.

American scientists have also discovered other properties of vitamin B3. In their opinion, it improves the ability of immune cells to kill Staphylococcus aureus bacteria (golden staph). Under the influence of vitamin B3, the number of neutrophils increases - white blood cells that can kill and absorb harmful bacteria. Probably certain antimicrobial genes are "turned on".

Niacin can help protect skin cells from sun damage. Niacin helps in treating acne and also improves skin elasticity.

Bissett DL, Oblong JE, Berge CA. **Niacinamide: A B vitamin that improves aging facial skin appearance.** Dermatol Surg. 2005 Jul;31(7 Pt 2):860-5; discussion 865. doi: 10.1111/ j.1524-4725.2005.31732. PMID: 16029679.

When applied to the skin, it reduces fine wrinkles, redness and discoloration.

It can help reduce oxidative stress and inflammation, both of which are involved in atherosclerosis.

Duggal JK, Singh M, Attri N, Singh PP, Ahmed N, Pahwa S, Molnar J, Singh S, Khosla S, Arora R. **Effect of niacin therapy on cardiovascular outcomes in patients with coronary artery disease.** J Cardiovasc Pharmacol Ther. 2010 Jun;15(2):158-66. doi: 10.1177/1074248410361337. Epub 2010 Mar 5. PMID: 20208032.

Niacin therapy has been shown to reduce the risk of

stroke.

Vitamin B3 supplementation as NAD + plays a key protective role for brain cells in people with neuro-degenerative diseases.

Furthermore, high doses of vitamin B3 along with vitamin C can help manage schizophrenia. Isn't it also worth a try? Especially since many drugs for schizophrenia destroy the body.

Niacin can possibly lower the risk of type 1 diabetes in at-risk children.

Skyler JS. **Primary and secondary prevention of Type 1 diabetes.** Diabet Med. 2013;30(2):161-169. doi:10.1111/dme.12100

The researchers noted that vitamin B3 (niacin) increases the activity of the mitochondria in the nucleus accumbens - the area of the brain responsible for the sensation of pleasure - induces a reduction in anxiety levels in laboratory rats. In this way, the rodents become more self-confident and achieve greater success in the herd.

Severe niacin deficiency causes a condition called pellagra.

Daily Niacin Requirement:

For men: 16 mg and for women: 14 mg

High vitamin B3 foods per 100g:
- Beef liver (88% DV)
- Chicken breast: (59% DV)
- Tuna (138% DV)
- Light tuna, canned in oil: (53% DV)
- Beef: (33% DV)
- Smoked salmon: (32% DV)
- Peanuts: (19% DV)

VITAMIN B4 (CHOLINE)

Choline is an essential nutrient. Its insufficient amounts are produced in the liver. Although classified as vitamin B4, it is neither a vitamin nor a mineral.

Vitamin B4 plays a very important role in the body, especially in pregnant women. It is involved in the development of the brain and nervous system of the fetus.

Caudill MA, Strupp BJ, Muscalu L, Nevins JEH, Canfield RL. **Maternal choline supplementation during the third trimester of pregnancy improves infant information processing speed**: a randomized, double-blind, controlled feeding study. FASEB J. 2018 Apr;32(4):2172-2180. doi: 10.1096/fj.201700692RR. Epub 2018 Jan 5. PMID: 29217669; PMCID: PMC6988845.

In a clinical trial of 26 pregnant women, doubling the choline intake in the third trimester of pregnancy (to 930 mg / day) significantly improved cognition (information processing speed) in infants. Increased choline intake during the second trimester of pregnancy may also improve visual memory in children.

Mellott TJ, Follettie MT, Diesl V, Hill AA, Lopez-Coviella I, Blusztajn JK. **Prenatal choline availability modulates hippocampal and cerebral cortical gene expression.** FASEB J. 2007 May;21(7):1311-23. doi: 10.1096/fj.06-6597com. Epub 2007 Jan 30. PMID: 17264169.

"These data show that the prenatal supply of choline causes multiple modifications in the developmental patterns of expression of genes known to influence learning and memory (...)"

Zeisel SH. **Choline: critical role during fetal development and dietary requirements in adults.** Annu Rev Nutr. 2006;26:229-50. doi: 10.1146/annurev.nutr.26.061505.111156. PMID: 16848706; PMCID: PMC2441939.

For pregnant women:
- Supports the development of the brain and spinal cord (central nervous system) of the fetus and newborn.
- Reduces the risk of birth defects.

- Improves blood flow in the placenta.

Zeisel SH, da Costa KA. **Choline: an essential nutrient for public health.** Nutr Rev. 2009;67(11):615-623. doi:10.1111/j.1753-4887.2009.00246.x

Low choline intake may raise your risk of other pregnancy complications.
Choline is involved in creating and maintaining the proper structure of cells, controlling muscle function, respiratory system, heart function and brain work related to memory. This nutrient is required to make acetylcholine, an important neurotransmitter. According to research, choline influences the improvement of long-term memory. Several studies have shown that choline can help with bipolar disorder in children.

A diet high in Choline may reduce the risk of developing dementia and conditions associated with Alzheimer's disease.
Furthermore, choline is involved in the regulation of lipid metabolism.

Elsawy G, Abdelrahman O, Hamza A. **Effect of choline supplementation on rapid weight loss and biochemical variables among female taekwon-**

do and judo athletes. J Hum Kinet. 2014 Apr 9;40:77-82. doi: 10.2478/hukin-2014-0009. PMID: 25031675; PMCID: PMC4096089.

In a clinical trial involving 22 athletes, supplementation with choline (2 g daily for 7 days before a competition) lowered the body mass index (BMI) by 12% without any side effects.

Gao X, Wang Y, Randell E, Pedram P, Yi Y, Gulliver W, Sun G. **Higher Dietary Choline and Betaine Intakes Are Associated with Better Body Composition in the Adult Population of Newfoundland**, Canada. PLoS One. 2016 May 11;11(5):e0155403. doi: 10.1371/journal.pone.0155403. PMID: 27166611; PMCID: PMC4863971.

"Our findings indicate that high dietary choline and betaine intakes are significantly associated with favorable body composition in humans."
According to an observational study involving over 3,200 people, lower dietary choline intake was associated with weight gain and excess body fat.

Choline may support the proper condition of the circulatory system.

Millard HR, Musani SK, Dibaba DT, et al. **Dieta-**

ry choline and betaine; associations with sub-clinical markers of cardiovascular disease risk and incidence of CVD, coronary heart disease and stroke: the Jackson Heart Study. Eur J Nutr. 2018;57(1):51-60. doi:10.1007/s00394-016-1296-8

In nearly 4,000 African-American patients, higher choline intake lowered the risk of stroke.
It may also reduce the risk of some cancers.

Du YF, Luo WP, Lin FY, Lian ZQ, Mo XF, Yan B, Xu M, Huang WQ, Huang J, Zhang CX. **Dietary choline and betaine intake, choline-metabolising genetic polymorphisms and breast cancer risk**: a case-con trol study in China. Br J Nutr. 2016 Sep;116(6):961-8. doi: 10.1017/S0007114516002956. Epub 2016 Aug 4. PMID: 27488260.

Higher choline intake was associated with lower percentage of breast cancer.

Lu MS, Fang YJ, Pan ZZ, Zhong X, Zheng MC, Chen YM, Zhang CX. **Choline and beta-ine intake and colorectal cancer risk in Chinese population: a case-control study.** PLoS One. 2015 Mar 18;10(3):e0118661. doi: 10.1371/

journal.pone.0118661. PMID: 25785727; PMCID: PMC4364675.

"These results indicate that high intake of total choline is associated with a lower risk of colorectal cancer."
In a study of over 1,700 patients, the highest choline intake correlated with an almost two-fold lower percentage of colorectal cancer.
A high dietary intake of choline may be associated with a lower rate of breast or colorectal cancer, but studies have shown that it also has a higher rate of prostate cancer. These findings require further research.

Choline may help treat asthma.

Mehta AK, Singh BP, Arora N, Gaur SN. **Choline attenuates immune inflammation and suppresses oxidative stress in patients with asthma.** Immunobiology. 2010 Jul;215(7):527-34. doi: 10.1016/j.imbio.2009.09.004. Epub 2009 Nov 7. PMID: 19897276.

Six-month choline supplementation (1500 mg, 2x / day) brought significant symptom relief and reduced inflammation in 74 patients with asthma. In addition, in animal models of asthma, choline reduces inflammation and oxidative stress.

It positively influences the work of the liver.

Fischer LM, daCosta KA, Kwock L, et al. **Sex and menopausal status influence human dietary requirements for the nutrient choline.** Am J Clin Nutr. 2007;85(5):1275-1285. doi:10.1093/ajcn/85.5.1275

A study in 57 adults confirmed that low choline intake can cause fatty liver disease, especially in postmenopausal women. Choline supplementation can prevent and reverse fatty liver as well as increase cholesterol metabolism.

High choline foods per 100g:
- Beef liver (85% DV)
- Lean Chicken Breast (21% DV)
- Lean Pork Chops (16% DV)
- Eggs (53% DV)
- Beef - Skirt Steak (14% DV)
- Shrimp (25% DV)
- Navy Beans (8% DV)

VITAMIN B5 (PANTOTHENIC ACID)

The active form of pantothenic acid is coenzyme A. Pantothenic acid is necessary for the production of antibodies that protect the body against bacterial and viral infections, and also plays a significant role in the regeneration of skin, mucous membranes and tissues. It also inhibits excessive reactions of the immune system.

Vitamin B5 is a substance that is able to increase the level of GSH (glutathione) in the mitochondria. Pantothenic acid supports proper metabolism and is essential for the functioning of the liver.

Vitamin B5 exhibits the properties of accelerating wound healing, prevents the formation of wrinkles and prevents premature aging and graying. It supports the hair pigmentation process.

Petri H, Pierchalla P, Tronnier H. Die Wirksamkeit einer medikamentösen Therapie bei Haarstrukturschäden und diffusen Effluvien--vergleichende Doppelblindstudie [**The efficacy of drug therapy in**

structural lesions of the hair and in diffuse efflu-
vium--comparative double blind study]. Schweiz
Rundsch Med Prax. 1990 Nov 20;79(47):1457-62.
German. Erratum in: Schweiz Rundsch Med Prax
1991 Feb 5;80(6):125. PMID: 1709511.

It was proved in a double-blind clinical trial that
pantothenic acid improved the condition of the
hair and reduced hair loss.

Leung LH. **Pantothenic acid deficiency as the pathogenesis of acne vulga-
ris**. Med Hypotheses. 1995 Jun;44(6):490-2. doi:
10.1016/0306-9877(95)90512-x. PMID: 7476595.

Vitamin B5 deficiency increases the frequency and
severity of acne. Dietary supplements based on
pantothenic acid reduce the number of changes on
the skin of the face.
Vitamin B5 also participates in the synthesis of
cholesterol, steroid hormones (such as cortisol,
testosterone, estradiol, progesterone), neurotransmitters (serotonin, dopamine), as well as vitamin
A and vitamin D.

Rumberger JA, Napolitano J, Azumano I, Kamiya
T, Evans M. **Pantethine, a derivative of vitamin B (5) used as a nutritional supplement,
favorably alters low-density lipoprotein chole-**

sterol metabolism in low- to moderate-cardiovascular risk North American subjects: a triple-blinded placebo and diet-controlled investigation. Nutr Res. 2011 Aug;31(8):608-15. doi: 10.1016/j.nutres.2011.08.001. PMID: 21925346.

Supplementing pantethine daily (600 mg/day for 8 weeks, followed by 900 mg/day for another 8 weeks), reported a significant improvement of the lipid parameter profile in individuals at low-to-moderate risk of cardiovascular disease (CVD). It also helps lower high blood pressure and prevents heart failure.

General Practitioner Research Group. **Calcium pantothenate in arthritic conditions.** A report from the General Practitioner Research Group. Practitioner. 1980; 224(1340):208–211

Research has shown that 2,000 mg/day calcium pantothenate improved symptoms of rheumatoid arthritis.

High vitamin B5 foods per 100g:
- Beef liver (71% DV)
- Shiitake Mushrooms (72% DV)
- Salmon (38% DV)
- Avocados (28% DV)

- Lean Chicken Breast (32% DV) and in a chicken thigh (34% DV)
- Sunflower Seeds (141% DV)

Among the B vitamins, vitamin B5 is the most sensitive to external factors.

VITAMIN B6

Vitamin B6 is absorbed into the bloodstream from the digestive system - so we supply it to the body with food.

One of the most important roles that vitamin B6 plays in our body is the control of important enzymes responsible for the course of key biochemical processes. Vitamin B6 is a coenzyme of over 100 enzymes (i. e. a substance necessary for the proper functioning of these compounds). Recent studies suggest that vitamin B6 might help reduce the risk of late-life depression. This is partly because this vitamin is necessary for creating neurotransmitters that regulate emotions. Researchers also suspect that B6 helps with emotional symptoms related to PMS (premenstrual syndrome).

De Souza MC, Walker AF, Robinson PA, Bolland K. **A synergistic effect of a daily supplement for 1 month of 200 mg magnesium plus 50 mg vitamin B6 for the relief of anxiety-related premenstrual symptoms:** a randomized, double-blind, crossover study. J Womens Health Gend Based Med. 2000

Ma-r;9(2):131-9. doi: 10.1089/152460900318623.
PMID: 10746516.

Another small study found that 50 mg of vitamin B6 along with 200 mg of magnesium per day significantly reduced PMS symptoms.

Herrmann W, Lorenzl S, Obeid R. Hyperhomocysteinämie und B-Vitaminmangel bei neurologischen und psychiatrischen Erkrankungen--Aktueller Kenntnisstand und vorläufige Empfehlungen [**Review of the role of hyperhomocysteinemia and B-vitamin deficiency in neurological and psychiatric disorders--current evidence and preliminary recommendations**]. Fortschr Neurol Psychiatr. 2007 Sep;75(9):515-27. German. doi: 10.1055/s-2007-980112. PMID: 17729191.

Vitamin B6 may also play a role in decreasing high blood levels of the amino acid homocysteine.

Seshadri S, Beiser A, Selhub J, Jacques PF, Rosenberg IH, D'Agostino RB, Wilson PW, Wolf PA. **Plasma homocysteine as a risk factor for dementia and Alzheimer's disease.** N Engl J Med. 2002 Feb 14;346(7):476-83. doi: 10.1056/NEJMoa011613. PMID: 11844848.

High homocysteine blood levels may increase the risk of Alzheimer's.

Vitamin B6 is also essential for the production of hemoglobin (red blood pigment).

Mason DY, Emerson PM. **Primary acquired sideroblastic anaemia: response to treatment with pyridoxal-5-phosphate.** Br Med J. 1973;1(5850):389-390. doi:10.1136/bmj.1.5850.389

A case study in a 72-year-old woman with anemia due to low B6 found that treatment with the most active form of this vitamin improved symptoms.

Lin PT, Cheng CH, Liaw YP, Lee BJ, Lee TW, Huang YC. **Low pyridoxal 5'-phosphate is associated with increased risk of coronary artery disease.** Nutrition. 2006 Nov-Dec;22(11-12):1146-51. doi: 10.1016/j.nut.2006.08.013. Epub 2006 Oct 10. PMID: 17045461.

Vitamin B6 reduces heart disease risk. People with low levels of vitamin B6 in their blood are almost twice as likely to develop heart disease as people with high levels. Vitamin B6 is also regulating the level of cysteine in the body (excess cysteine can lead to the development of atherosclerosis).

Some studies have shown that vitamin B6 can help prevent various types of cancer.

It increases the body's immunity - participates in the formation of antibodies. By reducing inflammation it may also help reduce symptoms associated with rheumatoid arthritis.

High vitamin B6 foods per 100g:
- Salmon (56% DV) and 104% DV in a 6oz tuna fillet
- Beef liver (51% DV)
- Lean Chicken Breast (54% DV) and 108% DV in 6oz of ground turkey
- Lean Pork Chops (32% DV)
- Beef - Skirt Steak (28% DV)
- In 1 cup of spinach (26% DV)
- Bananas (22% DV)

After ingestion, it is absorbed from the gastrointestinal tract and stored mainly in the muscles and liver as pyridoxal phosphate.

VITAMIN B7 (BIOTIN)

The body cannot synthesize biotin, so it must be obtained from the diet regularly.

Said HM. **Cell and molecular aspects of human intestinal biotin absorption.** J Nutr. 2009;139(1):158-162. doi:10.3945/jn.10-8.092023

Biotin is involved in the growth and development of the body.

Zempleni J, Hassan YI, Wijeratne SS. **Biotin and biotinidase deficiency.** Expert Rev Endocrinol Metab. 2008 Nov 1;3(6):715-724. doi: 10.1586/17446651.3.6.715. PMID: 19727438; PMCID: PMC2726758.

Biotin has been shown to be important for a number of health factors, including supporting neurological function, stabilizing blood sugar levels, DNA stability, and hair, skin, and nail health.

León-Del-Río A. **Biotin-dependent regulation of**

gene expression in human cells. J Nutr Biochem. 2005 Jul;16(7):432-4. doi: 10.1016/j.jnutbio.2005.03.021. PMID: 15992685.

Biotin is involved in gluconeogenesis - the synthesis of glucose from sources other than carbohydrates. Vitamin B7, along with other B vitamins, is needed to convert the food you eat into usable energy that supports a healthy metabolism. Biotin assists enzymes that activate reactions that are important for the production of fatty acids. Moreover, biotin deficiency lowers heme synthesis and disrupts mitochondrial functions. Inadequate levels of biotin in the body can slow down the metabolism, leading to fatigue, digestive problems and weight gain.

Marshall MW, Kliman PG, Washington VA, Mackin JF, Weinland BT. **Effects of biotin on lipids and other constituents of plasma of healthy men and women.** Artery. 1980;7(4):330-51. PMID: 7011260.

Vitamin B7 affects the lipid profile, which is crucial for the health of the heart and blood vessels. When combined with chromium, biotin can help reduce risk factors for heart disease.

Biotin is necessary for the formation of the myelin sheath, the substance that surrounds the nerves and helps conduct nerve impulses. Deficiency can lead to seizures, incoordination, difficulty in learning, hallucinations, depression and lethargy. Supplementation alleviates these conditions. For example, multiple sclerosis is a disorder characterized by damage to the myelin sheaths.

Sedel F, Papeix C, Bellanger A, Touitou V, Lebrun-Frenay C, Galanaud D, Gout O, Lyon-Caen O, Tourbah A. **High doses of biotin in chronic progressive multiple sclerosis**: a pilot study. Mult Scler Relat Disord. 2015 Mar;4(2):159-69. doi: 10.1016/ j.msard.2015.01.005. Epub 2015 Jan 24. PMID: 25787192.

Some studies have shown that high-dose biotin treatment has been able to reverse the progression of multiple sclerosis and improve symptoms.

Daily biotin supplementation reduced fasting blood sugar by an average of about 45% in patients with type 2 diabetes.

Lazo de la Vega-Monroy ML, Larrieta E, German MS, Baez-Saldana A, Fernandez-Mejia C. **Effects of biotin supplementation in the diet on insulin secretion, islet gene expression, glucose homeostasis and beta-cell proportion.** J Nutr Biochem. 2013 Jan;24(1):169-77. doi: 10.1016/

j.jnutbio.2012.03.020. Epub 2012 Jul 25. PMID: 22841397.

Biotin may be crucial in prevention and treatment of diabetes. Vitamin B7 increases insulin production and glucose uptake in muscle cells.
Biotin supports immunity, inhibits inflammation and can soothe allergic disorders.

Messaritakis J, Kattamis C, Karabula C, Matsaniotis N. **Generalized seborrhoeic dermatitis.** Clinical and therapeutic data of 25 patients. Arch Dis Child. 1975 Nov;50(11):871-4. doi: 10.1136/adc.50.11.871. PMID: 129036; PMCID: PMC1545716.

Biotin deficiency is associated with a number of skin diseases, including seborrheic dermatitis and eczema. Hair loss and nail brittleness may also occur.

The daily dose for adult men and women over 19 years of age is 30 µg / day.
High biotin foods per 100g
- Eggs (66% DV)
- Sunflower seeds (50% DV)
- Cooked chicken liver (613% DV)
- Cooked beef liver (137% DV)

VITAMIN B9

Vitamin B9 is one of the essential nutrients found in nature in the form of folates. Folic acid plays a vital role in cellular metabolism and energy production. It helps in the synthesis of DNA and RNA and regulates the level of homocysteine. Folic acid and magnesium are necessary for the construction of ribonucleotides that make up DNA and RNA.

Joshi R, Adhikari S, Patro BS, Chattopadhyay S, Mukherjee T. **Free radical scavenging behavior of folic acid: evidence for possible antioxidant activity.** Free Radic Biol Med. 2001 Jun 15;30(12):1390-9. doi: 10.1016/s0891-5849(01)00543-3. PMID: 11390184.

Folic acid is an antioxidant and increases the activity of antioxidant enzymes, e. g. SOD and catalase.

Morris MS, Jacques PF, Rosenberg IH, Selhub J. **Folate and vitamin B-12 status in relation to anemia, macrocytosis, and cognitive impairment in older Americans in the age of folic acid fortification.** Am J Clin Nutr. 2007 Jan;85(1):193-200. doi:

10.1093/ajcn/85.1.193. PMID: 17209196; PMCID: PMC1828842.

Folic acid is essential for the replication and division of red blood cells.

de Bree A, van Mierlo LA, Draijer R. **Folic acid improves vascular reactivity in humans:** a meta-analysis of randomized controlled trials. Am J Clin Nutr. 2007 Sep;86(3):610-7. doi: 10.1093/ajcn/86.3.610. PMID: 17823424.

Supplementation with high doses of folic acid effectively reduces the level of homocysteine and improves the condition of the vessels in patients with coronary artery disease.
In addition, folic acid supports the work of the brain.

Reynolds EH. **Benefits and risks of folic acid to the nervous system.** J Neurol Neurosurg Psychiatry. 2002;72(5):567-571. doi:10.1136/jnnp.72.5.567

People with low levels of folic acid in the blood show a deterioration in cognitive functions. The research concerns especially the elderly, with epilepsy and mental diseases. It is most likely related to an increase in homocysteine levels.

Supports reproductive functions.

Young SS, Eskenazi B, Marchetti FM, Block G, Wyrobek AJ. **The association of folate, zinc and antioxidant intake with sperm aneuploidy in healthy non-smoking men**. Hum Reprod. 2008 May;23(5):1014-22. doi: 10.1093/humrep/den036. Epub 2008 Mar 19. PMID: 18353905.

More folate intake is associated with fewer abnormal sperm counts in men. Pregnant women should also take care of high levels of folic acid. Low levels of folic acid in pregnant women are associated with abnormal fetal development.

Wilson RD; GENETICS COMMITTEE; MOTHERISK. **Pre-conceptional vitamin/folic acid supplementation 2007: the use of folic acid in combination with a multivitamin supplement for the prevention of neural tube defects and other congenital anomalies**. J Obstet Gynaecol Can. 2007 Dec;29(12):1003-1013. English, French. doi: 10.1016/S1701-2163(16)32685-8. Erratum in: J Obstet Gynaecol Can. 2008 Mar;30(3):193. Goh, Ingrid [corrected to Goh, Y Ingrid]. PMID: 18053387.

Folic acid in combination with a multivitamin supplement has been associated with a decrease in specific birth defects. It may minimize the risk of congenital heart defects, cleft palate and other abnormalities in the prenatal period. Supplementation may also reduce the frequency of premature births in pregnant women.

Folic acid can help prevent certain types of cancer.

Tio M, Andrici J, Cox MR, Eslick GD. **Folate intake and the risk of upper gastrointestinal cancers**: a systematic review and meta-analysis. J Gastroenterol Hepatol. 2014 Feb;29(2):250-8. doi: 10.1111/jgh.12446. PMID: 24224911.

Taking folic acid may be associated with a lower risk of colon cancer, esophagus, ovary, pancreas, and breast cancer. Low dietary intake of folate may increase the risk of developing breast cancer, particularly for women who drink alcohol.

It is also important that, along with vitamin K1, it participates in the synthesis of prothrombin, i. e. a substance responsible for blood clotting.

High vitamin B9 foods per 100g
- Green Soybeans (78% DV)
- Beef liver (65% DV)
- Lentils (45% DV) and in 1 cup of roman beans

(92% DV)
- Asparagus (37% DV)
- Spinach (37% DV)
- Broccoli (27% DV)
- Avocados (20% DV)
- Lettuce (34% DV)

VITAMIN B12 (COBALAMIN)

It is a vitamin produced with the participation of microorganisms. Since the body cannot produce it on its own, we must provide it with food. Vitamin B12 is stored in the liver. Vitamin B12 has an extremely versatile effect on the human body.

Green R, Datta Mitra A. **Megaloblastic Anemias: Nutritional and Other Causes.** Med Clin North Am. 2017 Mar;101(2):297-317. doi: 10.1016/j.mcna.2016.09.013. Epub 2016 Dec 14. PMID: 28189172.

Vitamin B12 is involved in the formation of red blood cells and the prevention of anemia. It is needed for the proper maturation of erythrocytes and maintaining their proper level.

Vitamin B12 protects mitochondria against oxidative stress and supports their proper functioning.

Lee YJ, Wang MY, Lin MC, Lin PT. **Associations between **Vitamin B-12 Status and Oxidative Stress and Inflammation in Diabetic Vegetarians and Omnivores**. Nutrients. 2016;8(3):118. Published 2016 Feb 26. doi:10.3390/nu8030118

The activity of antioxidant enzymes that protect against oxidative stress is higher in people with higher levels of vitamin B12 than in those who are deficient. During a vitamin B12 deficiency, the level of a certain substance rises and its excess causes damage to the mitochondria.

Vitamin B12 affects the health of the cardiovascular system. It lowers the level of homocysteine and for this reason it helps to protect against heart disease such as heart attack or stroke. Whereas vitamin B12 deficiency causes an increase in homocysteine levels. Important? Very.

Vitamin B12 also has an analgesic effect. The most effective form of vitamin B12 for this purpose is methylcobalamin. It concerns pains of nervous origin.

Yamashiki M, Nishimura A, Kosaka Y. **Effects of methylcobalamin (vitamin B12) on in vitro cytokine production of peripheral blood mononuclear cells.** J Clin Lab Immunol. 1992;37(4):173-82. PMID: 1339917.

Scientists think that methylcobalamin may help patients with rheumatoid arthritis.

Zhang M, Han W, Hu S, Xu H. **Methylcobalamin: a potential vitamin of pain killer.** Neural Plast. 2013;2013:424651. doi: 10.1155/2013/424651. Epub 2013 Dec 26. PMID: 24455309; PMCID: PMC3888748.

Methylcobalamin increases the speed of nerve impulse conduction, myelin regeneration, neuron regeneration and inhibits the transmission of peripheral pain.

Mauro GL, Martorana U, Cataldo P, Brancato G, Letizia G. **Vitamin B12 in low back pain:** a randomised, double-blind, placebo-controlled study. Eur Rev Med Pharmacol Sci. 2000 May-Jun;4(3):53-8. PMID: 11558625.

Watanabe T, Kaji R, Oka N, Bara W, Kimura J. **Ultra-high dose methylcobalamin promotes nerve regeneration in experimental acrylamide neuropathy.** J Neurol Sci. 1994 Apr;122(2):140-3. doi: 10.1016/0022-510x(94)90290-9. PMID: 8021696.

The efficacy and safety of the intramuscular injection of cobalamin was confirmed in relieving low back pain in patients with no signs of nutritional deficiency. It also helps relieve pain in mouth ulcers and neuropathies.

Hooshmand B, Solomon A, Kåreholt I, Rusanen M, Hänninen T, Leiviskä J, Winblad B, Laatikainen T, Soininen H, Kivipelto M. **Associations between serum homocysteine, holotranscobalamin, folate and cognition in the elderly: a longitudinal study.** J Intern Med. 2012 Feb;271(2):204-12. doi: 10.1111/j.1365-2796.2011.02484.x. Epub 2011 Dec 30. PMID: 22077644.

Research shows that taking vitamin B12 and folate improves brain performance. Folic acid and vitamin B12 deficiencies also contribute to brain degeneration. Supplementation with vitamins B6, B12 and folic acid improves speech and cognitive functions. The higher the deficiency of these ingredients, the faster the loss of mental abilities after 65 years of age occurs.

Bottiglieri T. **Folate, vitamin B12, and neuropsychiatric disorders**. Nutr Rev. 1996 Dec;54(12):382-90. doi: 10.1111/j.1753-4887.1996.tb03851.x. PMID: 9155210.

Vitamin B12 deficiency can cause a variety of neurological and psychiatric disorders. Due to its role in the health of the nervous system, it can be used to reduce the risk of Alzheimer's disease and dementia. Supplementation with vitamin B12 helps in reversing the effects of a previous vitamin B12 deficiency.

Honma K, Kohsaka M, Fukuda N, Morita N, Honma S. **Effects of vitamin B12 on plasma melatonin rhythm in humans: increased light sensitivity phase-advances the circadian clock?** Experientia. 1992 Aug 15;48(8):716-20. doi: 10.1007/BF02124286. PMID: 1516676.

Vitamin B12 supports proper sleep. It can improve the circadian rhythm and the effect of melatonin.

Coppen A, Bolander-Gouaille C. **Treatment of depression: time to consider folic acid and vitamin B12.** J Psychopharmacol. 2005 Jan;19(1):59-65. doi: 10.1177/0269881105048899. PMID: 15671130.

Vitamin B12 can help treat depression. Vitamin B12, along with folic acid, is essential for the production of SAM, which is vital for neurological function, stress management, and mood regulation. Researchers suggest, on the basis of current data, oral doses of both folic acid (800 microg daily) and vitamin B12 (1 mg daily).

Vitamin B12 contributes also to the proper condition of the skin. Helps with acne, inflammation, psoriasis and eczema (applied to the skin).

High vitamin B12 foods per 100g:
- Clams (4120% DV) and in 3 oz of oysters (1020% DV)
- Beef liver (1386% DV)
- Tuna (453% DV) and in 5 oz fillet of Atlantic herring (783% DV) and per cup of can-ned sardines (555% DV)
- Beef - Skirt Steak (314% DV)
- Swiss Cheese (128% DV)
- Eggs (46% DV)
For adult men and women over 14 years of age: 2.4 µg.
Vitamin B12 supplementation should always be accompanied by the intake of biotin and folic acid.

BRIEFLY ABOUT MINERALS AND ANTI-NUTRIENTS...

Vitamins alone without minerals are worthless. No fruit or vegetable can produce any mineral by itself. The mineral content of vegetables depends only on the quality of the soil. If the soil quality is poor, the quality of our vegetables is also poor.

Everyone knows a lot about calcium, but not about magnesium, zinc or selenium and especially iodine. Not to mention chromium or boron. It will be about it...

It is also good to remember about the so-called "anti-nutrients". These are substances that can block the absorption of certain elements.

Examples:

- Tannins (tea, legumes, coffee) - can decrease iron absorption.

- Phytic acid (whole grains, legumes, seeds, some nuts) - can decrease zinc, magnesium, iron and calcium absorption.

- Oxalates (tea, green leafy vegetables) - can decrease calcium absorption.

- Lectins (legumes e.g. beans, peanuts and whole grains) can decrease calcium, zinc, phosphorus and iron absorption.

- Glucosinolates (cruciferous vegetables e.g. cabbage, broccoli) - can decrease iodine absorption.

MAGNESIUM

It is an extremely important mineral for the proper functioning of the body.

Magnesium is the second (together with potassium) most vital intracellular cation, activating over 300 enzymes. Magnesium is essential for the production of ATP and for the proper synthesis of DNA, RNA and proteins. It is necessary for all living cells.

Yamanaka, R., Tabata, S., Shindo, Y. et al. **Mitochondrial Mg2+ homeostasis decides cellular energy metabolism and vulnerability to stress.** Sci Rep 6, 30027 (2016). https://doi.org/10.1038/srep30027

Insufficient amounts of magnesium can lead to decreased mitochondrial efficiency and increased production of reactive oxygen forms. This can result in a structural disruption of proteins and DNA. Magnesium deficiency strongly affects the production of ATP energy. ATP will not work for magnesium deficiencies.

Rock E, Astier C, Lab C, Vignon X, Gueux E, Motta C, Rayssiguier Y. **Dietary magnesium deficiency in rats enhances free radical production in skeletal muscle.** J Nutr. 1995 May;125(5):1205-10. doi: 10.1093/jn/125.5.1205. PMID: 7738680.

"These results strongly support the hypothesis that free radical-mediated injury could contribute to skeletal muscle lesions resulting from magnesium deficiency. "

In animals deficient in magnesium, there is a reduction in antioxidant capacity and mitochondrial dysfunction occurs. Magnesium therefore has antioxidant properties.

Nielsen FH. **Effects of magnesium depletion on inflammation in chronic disease.** Curr Opin Clin Nutr Metab Care. 2014 Nov;17(6):525-30. doi: 10.1097/MCO.0000000000000093. PMID: 25023192.

"Subclinical magnesium deficiency caused by low dietary intake often occurring in the population is a predisposing factor for chronic inflammatory stress that is conducive for chronic disease."

Low magnesium intake is associated with increased inflammation, contributing to the development of diseases.

Magnesium helps to keep the circulatory system in proper condition. Low levels of magnesium lead to abnormal blood pressure. Correct blood pressure depends on a balance between sodium and potassium as well as magnesium and calcium. Low levels of magnesium cause imbalance.

Houston M. **The role of magnesium in hypertension and cardiovascular disease.** J Clin Hypertens (Greenwich). 2011 Nov;13(11):843-7. doi: 10.1111/j.1751-7176.2011.00538.x. Epub 2011 Sep 26. PMID: 22051430.

Research shows that magnesium supplementation can help lower blood pressure. It is even more effective with combining magnesium with potassium and lowering sodium intake. The authors recommend 1000 mg of magnesium along with 4.7 g of potassium and <1.5 g of sodium. It also works with blood pressure medications.

The relationship between magnesium and calcium is very important. Magnesium is a calcium blocker. It removes calcium from the blood stream and, importantly, removes intracellular calicum. Such calcium in cells can lead to oxidation. Studies show that intracellular calcium levels are always elevated when intracellular oxidative stress is also elevated. Hence, the reduction of the intracellular calcium level through an increased supply of magnesium leads to an improvement in many diseases.

Rosique-Esteban N, Guasch-Ferré M, Hernández-Alonso P, Salas-Salvadó J. **Dietary Magnesium and Cardiovascular Disease**: A Review with Emphasis in Epidemiological Studies. Nutrients. 2018 Feb 1;10(2):168. doi: 10.3390/nu10020168. PMID: 29389872; PMCID: PMC5852744.

It has been estimated that increased consumption of magnesium-rich foods reduces the risk of cardiovascular death by 28%.

Nicola Veronese, Linda Berton, Sara Carraro, Francesco Bolzetta, Marina De Rui, Egle Perissinotto, Elena Debora Toffanello, Giulia Bano, Simona Pizzato, Fabrizia Miotto, Alessandra Coin, Enzo Manzato, Giuseppe Sergi, **Effect of oral magnesium supplementation on physical performance in healthy elderly women involved in a weekly exercise program**: a randomized controlled trial, The American Journal of Clinical Nutrition, Volume 100, Issue 3, September 2014, Pages 974–981, https://doi.org/10.3945/ajcn.113.080168

"Daily magnesium oxide supplementation for 12 wk seems to improve physical performance in healthy elderly women."

Magnesium deficiency can also reduce physical performance. It is essential for the proper functioning of the muscles, both at rest and during exercise.

Kass LS, Poeira F. **The effect of acute vs chronic magnesium supplementation on exercise and recovery on resistance exercise, blood pressure and total peripheral resistance on normotensive adults.** J Int Soc Sports Nutr. 2015 Apr 24;12:19. doi: 10.1186/s12970-015-0081-z. Erratum in: J Int Soc Sports Nutr. 2018 Jul 25;15(1):36. PMID: 25945079; PMCID: PMC4419474.

Magnesium supplementation had a positive effect on the results of endurance training. And magnesium supplements prevent or delay age-related decline in physical performance.

Magnesium affects bone health. It is needed for the activity and proper metabolism of vitamin D, which is essential for bone health. Low magnesium intake is associated with decreased bone mineral density and promotes osteoporosis.

Orchard TS, Larson JC, Alghothani N, Bout-Tabaku S, Cauley JA, Chen Z, LaCroix AZ, Wactawski-Wende J, Jackson RD. **Magnesium intake, bone mineral density, and fractures**: results from the Women's Health Initiative Observational Study. Am J Clin

Nutr. 2014 Apr;99(4):926-33. doi: 10.3945/ajcn. 113.067488. Epub 2014 Feb 5. PMID: 24500155; PMCID: PMC3953885.

In postmenopausal women, low magnesium intake correlated with faster bone loss or lower bone mineral density. However, an excess of magnesium can lead to defects in mineralization.

Magnesium reduces the risk of diabetes and insulin resistance. So maybe it is worth paying more attention to this element?

Chan KH, Chacko SA, Song Y, et al. **Genetic variations in magnesium-related ion channels may affect diabetes risk among African American and Hispanic American women**. J Nutr. 2015;145(3):418-424. doi:10.3945/jn.114.203489

Higher magnesium intake was associated with a lower risk of type 2 diabetes and metabolic disorders. Low magnesium levels increase the chances of developing insulin resistance.

Larsson SC, Wolk A. **Magnesium intake and risk of type 2 diabetes**: a meta-analysis. J Intern Med. 2007 Aug;262(2):208-14. doi: 10.1111/ j.1365-2796.2007.01840.x. PMID: 17645588.

Increased consumption of magnesium-rich foods may reduce the risk of type 2 diabetes. Insulin sensitivity and elevated blood sugar levels can be improved by increasing your magnesium intake.

Hanje AJ, Fortune B, Song M, Hill D, McClain C. **The use of selected nutrition supplements and complementary and alternative medicine in liver disease.** Nutr Clin Pract.2006;21(3):255-272. doi:10.1177/0115426506021003255

Low levels of magnesium are one of the causes of liver diseases, especially non-alcoholic fatty liver disease.

Magnesium is needed during pregnancy.

Hovdenak N, Haram K. **Influence of mineral and vitamin supplements on pregnancy outcome**. Eur J Obstet Gynecol Reprod Biol. 2012 Oct;164(2):127-32. doi: 10.1016/j.ejogrb.2012.06.020. Epub 2012 Jul 6. PMID: 22771225.

"(Mg) deficiency may cause hematological and teratogenic damage."
Magnesium deficiency in pregnancy may cause

malformations in the fetus.

Magnesium can help protect against cancer. Magnesium deficiency exacerbates chronic inflammation and may play a significant role in cancer. Middle-aged men with higher serum magnesium levels had a 50% lower risk of dying from cancer than those with low serum magnesium levels.

Dibaba D, Xun P, Yokota K, White E, He K. **Magnesium intake and incidence of pancreatic cancer**: the VITamins and Lifestyle study. Br J Cancer. 2015 Dec 1;113(11):1615-21. doi: 10.1038/bjc.2015.382. Epub 2015 Nov 10. PMID: 26554653; PMCID: PMC4705892.

"Magnesium intake may be beneficial in terms of primary prevention of pancreatic cancer."

Magnesium can help treat headaches and migraines. Significantly lowered serum magnesium levels have been observed in people who suffer from migraines and headache. A high dose (600 mg) of oral magnesium daily for 12 weeks significantly reduced the incidence of headaches by 41.6% of respondents, and also reduced the severity and duration of acute pain attacks.

Cox IM, Campbell MJ, Dowson D. **Red blood cell magnesium and chronic fatigue syndrome.**

Lancet. 1991 Mar 30;337(8744):757-60. doi: 10.1016/0140-6736(91)91371-z. PMID: 1672392.

Magnesium relieves chronic fatigue syndrome. Half of the patients with chronic fatigue syndrome suffered from magnesium deficiency during the observation period. It has also been found that obsessive disorder patients have also lower levels of magnesium.

Research suggests that magnesium deficiency contributes to the aggravation of anxiety.

Singewald N, Sinner C, Hetzenauer A, Sartori SB, Murck H. **Magnesium-deficient diet alters depression- and anxiety-related behavior in mice--influence of desipramine and Hypericum perforatum extract**. Neuropharmacology. 2004 Dec;47(8):1189-97. doi: 10.1016/j.neuropharm.2004.08.010. PMID: 15567428.

Low levels of magnesium are associated with increased symptoms of depression in several different age groups and ethnic populations. Magnesium supplementation has been associated with an improvement in symptoms of severe depression.

Severe stress increases the loss of magnesium. Mild magnesium deficiency often has no specific symptoms. According to Dr. Thomas Levy , 80-90% of people are deficient.

Overdosing of magnesium is not common as the kidneys excrete excess magnesium.

For women and men aged 19-30: 310 - 400 and mg / day.

In adults over 30 years of age 320 and 420 mg / day.

High magnesium foods per 100g:

- Pumpkin Seeds (131% DV)
- Spinach (21% DV)
- Tuna (15% DV)
- Almonds (64% DV)
- Dark Chocolate with about 85% cocoa (54% DV)
- Avocados (7% DV) and Lima Beans (18% DV)

POTASSIUM

Potassium is an essential mineral for the proper functioning of all living cells. Most of the potassium in the body is found inside cells, especially in the cells of muscles, bones, liver and red blood cells.

The main functions of potassium are to maintain the potential of the cell membrane and regulate the fluids in the cell as well as activate many enzymes and participate in the metabolism of carbohydrates and proteins.

Potassium affects the proper functioning of the mitochondria and the production of energy.

Potassium has an antioxidant effect. The increase in potassium levels blocks the excessive production of reactive oxygen species by white blood cells.

Ando K, Matsui H, Fujita M, Fujita T. **Protective effect of dietary potassium against cardiovascular damage in salt-sensitive hypertension: possible role of its antioxidant action.** Curr Vasc Pharmacol. 2010 Jan;8(1):59-63. doi: 10.2174/1570161107-90226561. PMID: 19485915.

Thus, it supports the circulatory system.

Wen W, Wan Z, Ren K, Zhou D, Gao Q, Wu Y, Wang L, Yuan Z, Zhou J. **Potassium supplementation inhibits IL-17A production induced by salt loading in human T lymphocytes via p38/MAPK-SGK1 pathway.** Exp Mol Pathol. 2016 Jun;100(3):370-7. doi: 10.1016/j.yexmp.2016.03.009. Epub 2016 Mar 25. PMID: 27020669.

Potassium supplementation prevents the development of autoimmune and inflammatory diseases.

Potassium lowers blood pressure.

Aburto NJ, Hanson S, Gutierrez H, Hooper L, Elliott P, Cappuccio FP. **Effect of increased potassium intake on cardiovascular risk factors and disease**: systematic review and meta-analyses. BMJ. 2013 Apr 3;346:f1378. doi: 10.1136/bmj.f1378. PMID: 23558164; PMCID: PMC4816263.

"High quality evidence shows that increased potassium intake reduces blood pressure in people with hypertension (...)". Moreover: "Higher potassium intake was associated with a 24% lower risk of stroke". Isn't it worth trying potassium over chemical antihypertensives with a huge number of side effects?

He FJ, MacGregor GA. Fortnightly review: **Beneficial effects of potassium.** BMJ. 2001 Sep 1;323(7311):497-501. doi: 10.1136/ bmj.323.7311.497. PMID: 11532846; PMCID: PMC1121081.

However, high potassium intake does not lower blood pressure in people with normal blood pressure.
It may lower blood pressure in hypertensive patients who consume a lot of sodium.

Siani A, Strazzullo P, Giacco A, Pacioni D, Celentano E, Mancini M. **Increasing the dietary potassium intake reduces the need for antihypertensive medication**. Ann Intern Med. 1991 Nov 15;115(10):753-9. doi: 10.7326/0003-4819-115-10-753. PMID: 1929022.

"Increasing the dietary potassium intake from natural foods is a feasible and effective measure to reduce antihypertensive drug treatment."
In many hypertensive patients on a potassium-rich diet, blood pressure normalized without the need for pharmacotherapy.

Castro H, Raij L. **Potassium in hypertension and cardiovascular disease**. Semin Nephrol. 2013 May;33(3):277-89. doi: 10.1016/j.semnephrol.2013.04.008. PMID: 23953805.

The balance between potassium and sodium is more strongly associated with an increased risk of cardiovascular disease than sodium or potassium consumption alone.
Research also suggests that increased potassium intake may protect against stroke.

D'Elia L, Barba G, Cappuccio FP, Strazzullo P. **Potassium intake, stroke, and cardiovascular disease a meta-analysis of prospective studies**. J Am Coll Cardiol. 2011 Mar 8;57(10):1210-9. doi: 10.1016/j.jacc.2010.09.070. PMID: 21371638.

One study found that increasing potassium intake by 1.64 g per day was associated with a 21% reduction in the risk of stroke.

Khaw KT, Barrett-Connor E. **Dietary potassium and stroke-associated mortality**. A 12-year prospective population study. N Engl J Med. 1987 Jan 29;316(5):235-40. doi: 10.1056/NEJM198701293160502. PMID: 3796701.

"These findings support the hypothesis that a high intake of potassium from food sources may protect against stroke-associated death." An increase in daily potassium intake of 10 mmol was associated with a 40% reduction in mortality in 859 people with a stroke for 12 years.

Potassium can benefit the kidneys.

Sharma S, McFann K, Chonchol M, de Boer IH, Kendrick J. **Association between dietary sodium and potassium intake with chronic kidney disease in US adults**: a cross-sectional study. Am J Nephrol. 2013;37(6):526-533. doi:10.1159/00035-1178

"Higher intake of sodium and potassium is associated with lower odds of CKD (chronic kidney disease) among US adults."
NHANES study of 13,917 participants suggests higher potassium intake is associated with lower incidence of chronic kidney disease. In addition, chronic potassium deficiencies cause functional and structural changes in the kidneys. With potassium deficiency, the risk of developing kidney stones may also increase.

Curhan GC, Willett WC, Speizer FE, Spiegelman D, Stampfer MJ. **Comparison of dietary calcium with** supplemental calcium and other nutrients as factors affecting the risk for kidney stones in women. Ann Intern Med. 1997 Apr 1;126(7):497-504. doi: 10.7326/0003-4819-126-7-199704010-00001. PMID: 9092314.

It has been shown that people taking higher doses of potassium had a 50% lower risk of developing kidney stones.
Potassium can reduce the risk of diabetes.

Rowe JW, Tobin JD, Rosa RM, Andres R. **Effect of experimental potassium deficiency on glucose and insulin metabolism**. Metabolism. 1980 Jun;29(6):498-502. doi: 10.1016/0026-0495(80)90074-8. PMID: 6991855.

"This study demonstrates that potassium depletion causes glucose intolerance, which is associated with impaired insulin secretion." It is important for the secretion of insulin from the pancreatic cells. Low blood potassium intake or levels are also associated with an increased risk of insulin resistance and diabetes.

Shin D, Joh HK, Kim KH, Park SM. **Benefits of potassium intake on metabolic syndrome**: The fourth Korean National Health and Nutrition

Examination Survey (KNHANES IV). Atherosclerosis. 2013 Sep;230(1):80-5. doi: 10.1016/j.atherosclerosis.2013.06.025. Epub 2013 Jul 12. PMID: 23958257.

"Our results reveal a significant inverse association between potassium intake and metabolic syndrome in adults."
Higher potassium intake reduces the risk of metabolic syndrome in men and women.

Potassium may help treat rheumatoid arthritis.

Rastmanesh R, Abargouei AS, Shadman Z, Ebrahimi AA, Weber CE. **A pilot study of potassium supplementation in the treatment of hypokalemic patients with rheumatoid arthritis**: a randomized, double-blinded, placebo-controlled trial. J Pain. 2008 Aug;9(8):722-31. doi: 10.1016/j.jpain.2008.03.006. Epub 2008 May 12. PMID: 18468955.

"The elevated serum cortisol and potassium values in the treatment group correlate negatively with patient's assessment of pain intensity, reflecting an anti-pain effect for potassium supplementation."
Potassium supplementation helps reduce joint pain caused by RA. In addition, patients with rheuma-

toid arthritis (RA) have significantly lower levels of potassium in the serum and in the body than healthy people. Higher potassium intake leads to increased levels of production and secretion of cortisol in the blood, which alleviates symptoms of rheumatoid arthritis. Nearly 44% of those who took 6,000 mg of potassium per day for 28 days reported a 33% reduction in the intensity of pain associated with arthritis.

Potassium reduces the risk of osteoporosis.

Macdonald HM, New SA, Fraser WD, Campbell MK, Reid DM. **Low dietary potassium intakes and high dietary estimates of net endogenous acid production are associated with low bone mineral density in premenopausal women and increased markers of bone resorption in postmenopausal women**. Am J Clin Nutr. 2005 Apr;81(4):923-33. doi: 10.1093/ajcn/81.4.923. PMID: 15817873.

A diet high in potassium can help prevent osteoporosis and improve bone mineral density.

Lemann J Jr, Pleuss JA, Gray RW, Hoffmann RG. **Potassium administration reduces and potassium deprivation increases urinary calcium excretion in healthy adults** [corrected]. Kidney Int. 1991 May;39(5):973-83. doi: 10.1038/ki.1991.123. Erratum in: Kidney Int 1991 Aug;40(2):388. PMID: 1648646.

Furthermore, potassium supplementation is associated with faster reconstruction and reduced bone degradation.

The recommended adult potassium intake is 4.7 g / day.
High potassium foods per 100g:
- Avocados (10% DV)
- Salmon (13% DV)
- Beet Greens (19% DV)
- White Beans (12% DV)
- Tomato (5% DV)
- 240 ml of coconut water (13% DV)

ZINC

Zinc is an antioxidant that reduces inflammation in the body. The correct level of this element affects the activity of antioxidant enzymes.

Joray ML, Yu TW, Ho E, et al. **Zinc supplementation reduced DNA breaks in Ethiopian women.** Nutr Res. 2015;35(1):49-55. doi:10.1016/j.nutres.2014.10.006

It has been shown that women taking zinc had fewer amounts of DNA damage from reactive oxygen species.

Fortes C, Agabiti N, Fano V, Pacifici R, Forastiere F, Virgili F, Zuccaro P, Perruci CA, Ebrahim S. **Zinc supplementation and plasma lipid peroxides in an elderly population.** Eur J Clin Nutr. 1997 Feb;51(2):97-101. doi: 10.1038/sj.ejcn.1600369. PMID: 9049568.

"Adequate zinc intake or supplementation could play an important role in the prevention and/ or modulation of diseases in the elderly people." A study in the elderly showed that zinc supplementation reduced the amount of harmful peroxides in the blood.

Rostan EF, DeBuys HV, Madey DL, Pinnell SR. **Evidence supporting zinc as an important antioxidant for skin.** Int J Dermatol. 2002 Sep;41(9):606-11. doi: 10.1046/j.1365-4362.2002.01567.x. PMID: 12358835.

The antioxidant effect of zinc also applies to the skin.

Prasad AS, Bao B, Beck FW, Sarkar FH. **Zinc-suppressed inflammatory cytokines by induction of A20-mediated inhibition of nuclear factor-κB**. Nutrition. 2011 Jul-Aug;27(7-8):816-23. doi: 10.1016/j.nut.2010.08.010. Epub 2010 Oct 29. PMID: 21035309.

The presence of zinc in a certain protein reduces the production of inflammatory cytokines and inhibits inflammation. The results were similar in the elderly (often zinc deficient).

Göransson K, Lidén S, Odsell L. **Oral zinc in acne vulgaris**: a clinical and methodological study. Acta Derm Venereol. 1978;58(5):443-8. PMID: 82356.

Morgan CI, Ledford JR, Zhou P, Page K. **Zinc supplementation alters airway inflammation and airway hyperresponsiveness to a common allergen**. J Inflamm (Lond). 2011;8:36. Published 2011 Dec 7. doi:10.1186/1476-9255-8-36

"(...) suggesting zinc supplementation as a potential treatment for asthmatics." Zinc is also effective in inflammation associated with diseases such as irritable bowel syndrome, acne and asthma.
It has a positive effect on autoimmune diseases and zinc deficiency is common in people with these diseases.

Simkin PA. **Oral zinc sulphate in rheumatoid arthritis.** Lancet. 1976 Sep 11;2(7985):539-42. doi: 10.1016/s0140-6736(76)91793-1. PMID: 60622.

Positive changes in the reduction of joint swelling, morning stiffness and after zinc supplementation were observed in patients with rheumatoid arthritis.

Maywald M, Rink L. **Zinc supplementation induces CD4+CD25+Foxp3+ antigen-specific regulatory T cells and suppresses IFN-γ production by upregulation of Foxp3 and KLF-10 and downregulation**

of IRF-1. Eur J Nutr. 2017 Aug;56(5):1859-1869. doi: 10.1007/s00394-016-1228-7. Epub 2016 Jun 3. PMID: 27260002.

"Thus, zinc can be seen as an auspicious tool for inducing tolerance in adverse immune reactions." Research shows that zinc can also suppress some unwanted immune responses.

It is crucial for the immune system.

Ibs KH, Rink L. **Zinc-altered immune function**. J Nutr. 2003 May;133(5 Suppl 1):1452S-6S. doi: 10.1093/jn/133.5.1452S. PMID: 12730441.

Zinc is essential for the proper functioning of many immune cells.

Keen CL, Gershwin ME. **Zinc deficiency and immune function**. Annu Rev Nutr. 1990;10:415-31. doi: 10.1146/annurev.nu.10.070190.002215. PMID: 2200472.

Deficiency of this element may lead to impaired immunity and increase the risk of bacterial, viral and parasitic infections. Who has ever heard of taking zinc for such infections? Again, not many.

Baum MK, Lai S, Sales S, Page JB, Campa A. **Randomized, controlled clinical trial of zinc supplementation to prevent immunological failure in HIV-infected adults**. Clin Infect Dis. 2010 Jun 15;50(12):1653-60. doi: 10.1086/652864. PMID: 20455705; PMCID: PMC2874106.

Studies in patients with HIV and low blood zinc levels indicate that long-term supplementation is associated with fewer infections and a lower risk of immune failure.

Prasad AS. **Zinc: role in immunity, oxidative stress and chronic inflammation.** Curr Opin Clin Nutr Metab Care. 2009 Nov;12(6):646-52. doi: 10.1097/MCO.0b013e3283312956. PMID: 19710611.

Gupta M, Mahajan VK, Mehta KS, Chauhan PS. **Zinc therapy in dermatology**: a review. Dermatol Res Pract. 2014;2014:709152. doi: 10.1155/2014/709152. Epub 2014 Jul 10. PMID: 25120566; PMCID: PMC4120804.

Prasad AS. Discovery of human zinc deficiency: **its impact on human health and disease.** Adv Nutr. 2013;4(2):176-190. Published 2013 Mar 1. doi:10.3945/an.112.003210

Beneficial effects of zinc supplementation have also been reported for human infectious diseases, including Shigella infection, tuberculosis, leishmaniasis, hepatitis C, the common cold and in acute diarrhea in children.

This element modulates the transmission of nerve signals in synapses.

Penland JG, Sandstead HH, Alcock NW, Dayal HH, Chen XC, Li JS, Zhao F, Yang JJ. A preliminary report: **effects of zinc and micronutrient repletion on growth and neuropsychological function of urban Chinese children.** J Am Coll Nutr. 1997 Jun;16(3):268-72. doi: 10.1080/07315724.1997.10718684. PMID: 9176834.

"The findings confirm the essentiality of zinc for growth of children, and show, for the first time, the essentiality of zinc for neuropsychological functions of children."

Study found that supplementation with zinc provides improved neuropsychological performance, particularly attention and reasoning skills. Zinc supplementation in infants and young children leads to increased activity and better mental development.

Aquilani R, Baiardi P, Scocchi M, Iadarola P, Verri M, Sessarego P, Boschi F, Pasini E, Pastoris O, Viglio S. **Normalization of zinc intake enhances neurological retrieval of patients suffering from ischemic strokes**. Nutr Neurosci. 2009 Oct;12(5):219-25. doi: 10.1179/147683009X423445. PMID: 19761652.

"The normalization of Zn2+ intake in stroke patients with low mineral intake may enhance neurological recovery."
Zinc also helps in patients with zinc deficiency who have had an ischemic stroke.

Zinc therapy in people with Alzheimer's may protect against cognitive decline by reducing the level of free copper in the blood (free copper can be toxic to the brain).
Zinc can reduce the symptoms of obsessive compulsive disorder. Zinc may also be helpful in the case of schizophrenia and hyperactivity and impulsivity in children with ADHD.
Zinc can help with autism. Autistic people have lower levels of zinc.

Russo AJ, Devito R. **Analysis of Copper and Zinc Plasma Concentration and the Efficacy of Zinc Therapy in Individuals with Asperger's Syn-**

drome, Pervasive Developmental Disorder Not
Otherwise Specified (PDD-NOS) and Autism.
Biomark Insights. 2011;6:127-133. doi:10.4137/
BMI.S7286

"Severity of symptoms decreased in autistic individuals following zinc and B-6 therapy with respect to awareness, receptive language, focus and attention, hyperactivity, tip toeing, eye contact, sound sensitivity, tactile sensitivity and seizures. None of the measured symptoms worsened after therapy."

Certain autistic symptoms improved after treatment with zinc and vitamin B6. In addition, researchers from the University of Auckland showed that zinc can help reverse changes in brain cells in people with autism.

Maes M, Mihaylova I, De Ruyter M. **Lower serum zinc in Chronic Fatigue Syndrome (CFS): relationships to immune dysfunctions and relevance for the oxidative stress status in CFS.** J Affect Disord. 2006 Feb;90(2-3):141-7. doi: 10.1016/j.jad.2005.11.002. Epub 2005 Dec 9. PMID: 16338007.

Zinc has been found to be effective in relieving symptoms of chronic fatigue syndrome due to its antioxidant and anti-inflammatory properties.

Saad K, El-Houfey AA, Abd El-Hamed MA, El-Asheer OM, Al-Atram AA, Tawfeek MS. **A randomized, double-blind, placebo-controlled clinical trial of the efficacy of treatment with zinc in children with intractable epilepsy.** Funct Neurol. 2015;30(3):181-185. doi:10.11138/fneur/2015.30.3.181

Zinc supplementation significantly reduces the frequency of seizures in treated children with epilepsy.
Zinc can also help with digestive diseases.

Skrovanek S, DiGuilio K, Bailey R, et al. **Zinc and gastrointestinal disease.** World J Gastrointest Pathophysiol. 2014;5(4):496-513. doi:10.4291/wjgp.v5.i4.496

"Zinc enhancement of gastrointestinal epithelial barrier function may figure prominently in its potential therapeutic action in several gastrointestinal diseases."
Zinc helps to seal the epithelium of the digestive tract and strengthens the protective barrier, which may play a significant therapeutic role in diseases of the digestive tract.

Sturniolo GC, Di Leo V, Ferronato A,

D'Odorico A, D'Incà R. **Zinc supplementation tightens "leaky gut" in Crohn's disease**. Inflamm Bowel Dis. 2001 May;7(2):94-8. doi: 10.1097/00054725-200105000-00003. PMID: 11383597.

In addition: "Our findings show that zinc supplementation can resolve permeability alterations in patients with Crohn's disease in remission. Improving intestinal barrier function may contribute to reduce the risk of relapse in Crohn's disease".

Zinc has a positive effect on the skin. Zinc deficiency delays the wound healing process. Furthermore, administration of zinc may accelerate the tissue healing process following surgery and burns.

Gupta M, Mahajan VK, Mehta KS, Chauhan PS. **Zinc therapy in dermatology: a review**. Dermatol Res Pract. 2014;2014:709152. doi: 10.1155/2014/709152. Epub 2014 Jul 10. PMID: 25120566; PMCID: PMC4120804.

The use of zinc is beneficial in many skin diseases and conditions, such as acne, rosacea, eczema, psoriasis and dandruff.

Verma KC, Saini AS, Dhamija SK. **Oral zinc sulphate therapy in acne vulgaris:** a double-blind trial. Acta Derm Venereol. 1980;60(4):337-40. doi:

10.2340/0001555560337340. PMID: 6163281.

People with acne vulgaris who took zinc orally had significant improvements in symptoms compared to those taking placebo.

Zinc can treat seborrheic dermatitis and dandruff (used for example as a shampoo with zinc). Studies have also shown that oral zinc supplementation has a protective effect against ultraviolet radiation.

Bhardwaj P, Rai DV, Garg ML. **Zinc as a nutritional approach to bone loss prevention in an ovariectomized rat model. Meno-pause.** 2013 Nov;20(11):1184-93. doi: 10.1097/GME.0b013e31828a7f4e. PMID: 23571522.

Due to its strengthening effect on the bones, zinc protects against many bone related diseases and complications.

Zinc improves insulin sensitivity.

Jansen J, Karges W, Rink L. **Zinc and diabetes--clinical links and molecular mechanisms.** J Nutr Biochem. 2009 Jun;20(6):399-417. doi: 10.1016/j.jnutbio.2009.01.009. PMID: 19442898.

Zinc activates insulin signaling pathways by binding to the insulin receptor. Zinc deficiency is also common in patients with type 2 diabetes.

Vashum KP, McEvoy M, Shi Z, Milton AH, Islam MR, Sibbritt D, Patterson A, Byles J, Loxton D, Attia J. **Is dietary zinc protective for type 2 diabetes? Results from the Australian longitudinal study on women's health.** BMC Endocr Disord. 2013 Oct 4;13:40. doi: 10.1186/1472-6823-13-40. PMID: 24093747; PMCID: PMC4015935

"Higher total dietary zinc intake and high zinc/iron ratio are associated with lower risk of type 2 diabetes in women."

Marreiro DN, Geloneze B, Tambascia MA, Lerário AC, Halpern A, Cozzolino SM. Participação do zinco na resistência à insulina [**Role of zinc in insulin resistance**]. Arq Bras Endocrinol Metabol. 2004 Apr;48(2):234-9. Portuguese. doi: 10.1590/s0004-27302004000200005. Epub 2004 Jul 7. PMID: 15640877.

"Regarding obesity and insulin resistance, alterations in zinc concentration and distribution in tissues, as well as improvement in sensitivity to insulin after supplementation with this element, have been detected."

Its deficiency can lead to increased insulin resistance. Additionally zinc supplementation may have beneficial effects on glycemic control.

Nishiyama S, Futagoishi-Suginohara Y, Matsukura M, Nakamura T, Higashi A, Shinohara M, Matsuda I. **Zinc supplementation alters thyroid hormone metabolism in disabled patients with zinc deficiency.** J Am Coll Nutr. 1994 Feb;13(1):62-7. doi: 10.1080/07315724.1994.10718373. PMID: 8157857.

It is important for the proper functioning of the thyroid gland.

Kralik A, Eder K, Kirchgessner M. **Influence of zinc and selenium deficiency on parameters relating to thyroid hormone metabolism.** Horm Metab Res. 1996 May;28(5):223-6. doi: 10.1055/s-2007-979169. PMID: 8738110.

Zinc deficiency affects the low level of the thyroid hormones triiodothyronine (T3) and free thyroxine (FT4) in the blood, even causing hypothyroidism.

Amin AI, Hegazy NM, Ibrahim KS, Mahdy-Abdallah H, Hammouda HA, Shaban EE. **Thyroid Hormone Indices in Computer Workers with Emphasis on the Role of Zinc Supplementation.** Open Access Maced J Med Sci. 2016;4(2):296-301. doi:10.3889/

oamjms.2016.041

"Improvement after supplementation suggests that zinc can ameliorate hazards of such radiation on thyroid hormone indices."

Zinc supplementation had a positive effect in reversing the harmful effects of radiation emitted by a computer monitor.

Zinc contributes to the proper blood clotting process.

Zinc is essential for the reproductive capacity of men. It participates in the synthesis of testosterone.

Dissanayake D, Wijesinghe P, Ratnasooriya W, Wimalasena S. **Relationship between seminal plasma zinc and semen quality in a subfertile population.** J Hum Reprod Sci. 2010;3(3):124-128. doi:10.4103/0974-1208.74153

"Count, motility, viability, pH and viscosity are affected by variations of seminal plasma zinc."

Higher levels of zinc in the body have a positive effect on the number of sperm, their mobility and viability.

Netter A, Hartoma R, Nahoul K. **Effect**

of zinc administration on plasma testosterone, dihydrotestosterone, and sperm
count. Arch Androl. 1981 Aug;7(1):69-73. doi:
10.3109/01485018109009378. PMID: 7271365.

In infertile men, zinc supplementation increased
sperm count, testosterone, and dihydrotestosterone (DHT). This had a positive effect on fertility.
Moreover, zinc supplementation may increase libi-
do and sexual performance in men with erectile
dysfunction.

Favier AE. **The role of zinc in reproduction. Hormonal mechanisms.** Biol Trace Elem Res. 1992 Jan-
Mar;32:363-82. doi: 10.1007/BF02784623. PMID:
1375078.

"Zinc supplementation has already proven beneficial in male sterility and in reducing complications
during pregnancy. "
Zinc deficiency can lead to problems with the functioning of the ovaries, menstrual disorders and
infertility.

Kashefi F, Khajehei M, Tabatabaeichehr M, Ala-
vinia M, Asili J. **Comparison of the effect of
ginger and zinc sulfate on primary dysmenor-
rhea**: a placebo-controlled randomized trial. Pain

Manag Nurs. 2014 Dec;15(4):826-33. doi: 10.1016/ j.pmn.2013.09.001. Epub 2014 Feb 20. PMID: 24559600.

Administration of zinc may be able to reduce the intensity and duration of menstrual pain in women.

Messalli EM, Schettino MT, Mainini G, Ercolano S, Fuschillo G, Falcone F, Esposito E, Di Donna MC, De Franciscis P, Torella M. **The possible role of zinc in the etiopathogenesis of endometriosis.** Clin Exp Obstet Gynecol. 2014;41(5):541-6. PMID: 25864256.

Additionally: "The results showed that serum zinc levels in women with endometriosis are decreased and this seems to actually confirm that this micro-element can possibly affect the multifactorial pathogenesis of the disease".

The recommended daily allowance of zinc (RDA) for women and men over 19 is: 8 mg and 11 mg. And in the case of pregnancy and lactation: 11 mg, 12 mg.
In the case of various ailments (viral, bacterial, etc.), this amount can be increased to 75-100 mg per day.

High Zinc foods per 100g:

- Oysters (555% DV)
- Beef (99% DV)
- Beef liver (35% DV)
- Lean Pork Chops (19% DV)
- Hemp Seeds (90% DV)
- Chicken Leg (19% DV)

COPPER

It is necessary for iron to bind to transferrin, and thus for the synthesis of hemoglobin. Deficiency can cause anemia and heart diseases.

Allen KG, Klevay LM. **Cholesterolemia and cardiovascular abnormalities in rats caused by copper deficiency. Atherosclerosis.** 1978 Jan;29(1):81-93. doi: 10.1016/0021-9150(78)90096-5. PMID: 629827.

"The hearts of copper deficient rats were hypertrophied with large areas of hemorrhage, inflammation and focal necrosis."
Copper affects the strength of blood vessels and the work of the heart.

Bügel S, Harper A, Rock E, O'Connor JM, Bonham MP, Strain JJ. **Effect of copper supplementation on indices of copper status and certain CVD risk markers in young healthy women.** Br J Nutr. 2005 Aug;94(2):231-6. doi: 10.1079/bjn20051470. PMID: 16115357.

Supplementation with 6 mg of copper for 4 weeks led to a 30% reduction in plasminogen activator inhibitor-1 (PAI-1) in young women, potentially reducing the risk of atherosclerosis.

Galhardi CM, Diniz YS, Rodrigues HG, Faine LA, Burneiko RC, Ribas BO, Novelli EL. **Beneficial effects of dietary copper supplementation on serum lipids and antioxidant defenses in rats**. Ann Nutr Metab. 2005 Sep-Oct;49(5):283-8. doi: 10.1159/000087294. Epub 2005 Aug 2. PMID: 16088091.

"Dietary Cu supplementation had beneficial effects on lipid profile by improving endogenous antioxidant defenses and decreasing the oxidative stress in vivo."

In rats, copper supplementation reduced blood triglyceride and LDL cholesterol levels.

Copper plays an important role in bone formation.

Strause L, Saltman P, Smith KT, Bracker M, Andon MB. **Spinal bone loss in postmenopausal women supplemented with calcium and trace minerals**. J Nutr. 1994 Jul;124(7):1060-4. doi: 10.1093/jn/124.7.1060. PMID: 8027856.

Copper supplementation in women at a dose of 3 mg daily for two years slowed the loss of bone mineral density that accompanies menopause.

Allen TM, Manoli A 2nd, LaMont RL. **Skeletal changes associated with copper deficiency.** Clin Orthop Relat Res. 1982 Aug;(168):206-10. PMID: 6809388.

Additionally, copper supplementation improves bone health in copper-deficient infants. In elderly patients with copper deficiency, copper also slows bone resorption.

Copper contributes to healthy skin. It affects the production of collagen and elastin.

Borkow G, Gabbay J, Dardik R, Eidelman AI, Lavie Y, Grunfeld Y, Ikher S, Huszar M, Zatcoff RC, Marikovsky M. **Molecular mechanisms of enhanced wound healing by copper oxide-impregnated dressings.** Wound Repair Regen. 2010 Mar-Apr;18(2):266-75. doi: 10.1111/j.1524-475X.2010.00573.x. Epub 2010 Mar 12. PMID: 20409151.

Copper in wound dressings has strong antimicrobial properties.

Caution should be exercised when taking copper supplementation because its excess is toxic. In the case of copper deficiency confirmed by medical examination, the recommended daily dose of this element is 1 to 5 mg.

High copper foods per 100g:
- Beef liver (714% DV)
- Oysters (493% DV)
- Shiitake Mushrooms (100% DV)
- Firm Tofu (42% DV)
- Sesame Seeds (274% DV)
- Cashews (247% DV)
- Salmon (36% DV)
- Dark Chocolate about 70-85% Cocoa (196% DV)

SELENIUM

Selenium is an essential mineral needed for optimal health.

Sun JY, Hou YJ, Fu XY, et al. **Selenium-Containing Protein From Selenium-Enriched Spirulina platensis Attenuates Cisplatin-Induced Apoptosis in MC3T3-E1 Mouse Preosteoblast by Inhibiting Mitochondrial Dysfunction and ROS-Mediated Oxidative Damage**. Front Physiol. 2019;9:1907. Published 2019 Jan 9. doi:10.3389/fphys.2018.01907

Selenium activates powerful antioxidant enzymes that protect cells and mitochondria against free radicals. Its protective mechanism is based on influencing glutathione - a powerful antioxidant.
Selenium deficiency and reduced glutathione peroxidase activity intensify the oxidation of lipids present in the membranes of the mitochondria, which intensifies oxidative stress and inflammation.

Duntas LH. **Selenium and inflammation: underlying anti-inflammatory mechanisms**. Horm

Metab Res. 2009 Jun;41(6):443-7. doi: 10.1055/ s-0029-1220724. Epub 2009 May 5. PMID: 19418416.

"This review evaluates some apparently key mechanisms of the anti-inflammatory action of selenium and advocates Se supplementation as a modulator of inflammatory response in infectious and autoimmune disease."
It inhibits the production of pro-inflammatory cytokines. Adequate intake of selenium raises the level of selenoproteins, which are helpful in lowering the inflammatory marker CRP.

Selenium is crucial for immunity.
Selenium deficiency weakens the body's normal immune response. Increased selenium intake stimulates the immune system, even in people who are not deficient.

Steinbrenner H, Al-Quraishy S, Dkhil MA, Wunderlich F, Sies H. **Dietary selenium in adjuvant therapy of viral and bacterial infections.** *Adv Nutr.* 2015;6(1):73-82. Published 2015 Jan 15. doi:10.3945/an.114.007575

"Dietary multimicronutrient supplements containing selenium up to 200 μg/d have potential as safe, inexpensive, and widely available adjuvant therapy in viral infections (e. g., HIV, IAV) as well as in coinfections by HIV and *M. tuberculosis* to support the chemotherapy and/or to improve fitness and quality of life of the patients (…)"

Lymphocytes of people who replenished selenium (200 µg / day) were more active and effective in destroying pathogens and cancer cells. It also helps in the fight against HIV. Selenium deficiency is associated with the development of viral infections. In people with selenium deficiency, even dormant and inactive viruses can become a threat. This is vital because knowledge of this element is almost nonexistent.

Selenium is important for the functioning of the thyroid gland. The thyroid gland also stores the most selenium.

Mara Ventura, Miguel Melo, Francisco Carrilho, **"Selenium and Thyroid Disease: From Pathophysiology to Treatment"**, International Journal of Endocrinology, vol. 2017, Article ID 1297658, 9 pages, 2017. https://doi.org/10.1155/2017/1297658

Selenium is essential for the production of the thyroid hormone T3 and the conversion of T4 to T3.

Toulis KA, Anastasilakis AD, Tzellos TG, Goulis

DG, Kouvelas D. **Selenium supplementation in the treatment of Hashimoto's thyroiditis:** a systematic review and a meta-analysis. Thyroid. 2010 Oct;20(10):1163-73. doi: 10.1089/thy.2009.0351. PMID: 20883174.

In clinical trials, selenium improved the mood and general well-being of people suffering from Hashimoto's.

Gärtner R, Gasnier BC, Dietrich JW, Krebs B, Angstwurm MW. **Selenium supplementation in patients with autoimmune thyroiditis decreases thyroid peroxidase antibodies concentrations.** J Clin Endocrinol Metab. 2002 Apr;87(4):1687-91. doi: 10.1210/jcem.87.4.8421. PMID: 11932302.

"We conclude that selenium substitution may improve the inflammatory activity in patients with autoimmune thyroiditis, especially in those with high activity."
In Hashimoto's patients with high levels of anti-TPO antibodies, selenium supplementation lowered their level and improved the structure of the thyroid gland.

Reid SM, Middleton P, Cossich MC, Crowther CA. **Interventions for clinical and subclinical hypothyroidism in pregnancy**. Cochrane Database Syst Rev. 2010 Jul 7;(7):CD007752. doi: 10.1002/14651858.CD007752.pub2. Update in: Cochrane Database Syst Rev. 2013;5:CD007752. PMID: 20614463.

In a study of 314 pregnant women, lower blood levels of selenium were associated with decreased thyroid function and thyroid damage.

Selenium supports fertility and reproductive health.

Barrington JW, Lindsay P, James D, Smith S, Roberts A. **Selenium deficiency and miscarriage: a possible link**? Br J Obstet Gynaecol. 1996 Feb;103(2):130-2. doi: 10.1111/j.1471-0528.1996.tb09663.x. PMID: 8616128.

"A reduction in serum selenium normally occurs in the first trimester of pregnancies that progress to term. However, a further statistically highly significant decrease in serum selenium was observed in those women who miscarried."

In women, an adequate level of selenium is especially important in the first stage of pregnancy. Women who miscarried had lower levels of selenium in their blood. Therefore, it is worth controlling the level of this element at this time.

Men also need selenium for the production of sperm and testosterone.

Scott R, MacPherson A, Yates RW, Hussain B, Dixon J. **The effect of oral selenium supplementation on human sperm motility.** Br J Urol. 1998 Jul;82(1):76-80. doi: 10.1046/ j.1464-410x.1998.00683.x. PMID: 9698665.

"This trial confirms the result of an earlier study, that selenium supplementation in subfertile men with low selenium status can improve sperm motility and the chance of successful conception."

In a study on infertile men, selenium supplements significantly increased sperm motility within 3 months and 11% of men achieved paternity.

Selenium affects the cells of the nervous system and neurotransmitters.

Cardoso BR, Cominetti C, Cozzolino SM. **Importance and management of micronutrient deficiencies in patients with Alzheimer's disease**. Clin Interv Aging. 2013;8:531-542. doi:10.2147/CIA.S27983

Low selenium levels are associated with cognitive decline and memory problems. Patients with Alzheimer's disease had 60% lower levels of selenium in the brain compared to healthy people.

Berr C, Akbaraly T, Arnaud J, Hininger I, Roussel AM, Barberger Gateau P. **Increased selenium intake in elderly high fish consumers may account for health benefits previously ascribed to omega-3 fatty acids.** J Nutr Health Aging. 2009 Jan;13(1):14-8. doi: 10.1007/s12603-009-0003-3. PMID: 19151902.

"The observed health benefits of fish consumption in the elderly could be related not only to the increase in omega3 FA intake but also to other nutrients such as selenium."

Selenium works in synergy with omega-3 fatty acids, preventing their breakdown and increasing their beneficial effect on cognition. So it is important for protecting the brain.

Benton D, Cook R. **The impact of selenium supplementation on mood.** Biol Psychiatry. 1991 Jun 1;29(11):1092-8. doi: 10.1016/0006-3223(91)90251-g. PMID: 1873372.

Low selenium levels are also correlated with depression, anxiety and confusion.

"The lower the level of selenium in the diet the more reports of anxiety, depression, and tiredness, decreased following 5 weeks of selenium therapy."

So selenium affects also a more positive mood. It had a similar effect on hospitalized elderly cancer and / or HIV patients.

Selenium can help prevent cancer and soothe the effects of chemotherapy. Research indicates that low selenium levels are associated with an increased risk of cancer and death.

Fritz H, Kennedy D, Fergusson D, et al. **Selenium and lung cancer:** a systematic review and meta analysis. PLoS One.2011;6(11):e26259. doi:10.1371/journal.pone.0026259

Peters U, Takata Y. **Selenium and the prevention of prostate and colorectal cancer.** Mol Nutr Food Res. 2008;52(11):1261-1272. doi:10.1002/mnfr.200800103

Increased but non-toxic levels of selenium have been shown to reduce the risk of colon, prostate and lung cancer. In addition, another study found that also selenium reduced the risk of death over eight to ten years in people who had lung, colon and prostate cancer.

Combs GF Jr, Clark LC, Turnbull BW. **Reduction of cancer risk with an oral supplement of selenium.**

Biomed Environ Sci. 1997 Sep;10(2-3):227-34. PMID: 9315315.

The use of selenium supplementation in the amount of only 200 μg a day reduced mortality by 21% and the incidence of prostate cancer by 65%.

Cassidy PB, Fain HD, Cassidy JP Jr, et al. **Selenium for the prevention of cutaneous melanoma.** Nutrients. 2013;5(3):725-749. Published 2013 Mar 7. doi:10.3390/nu5030725

In another study, supplementation also increased the survival of people with skin cancer by 50%.

The form of selenium is also very important. Sodium selenite seems to be the most effective. The daily selenium requirement is approximately 55 μg per day for adults.

High Selenium Foods per 100g:

- Brazil Nuts (3485% DV) and in 1oz of sunflower seeds (41% DV)
- Tuna (197% DV)
- Shellfish (280% DV)
- Lean Pork Chops (86% DV)
- Beef (Skirt Steak) (65% DV)
- Beef Liver (52% DV)
- Shrimp (90% DV)
- Shiitake Mushrooms (45% DV)
- Lean Chicken Breast (58% DV)

IRON

Iron is another very important mineral necessary for the functioning of most living organisms. It is a catalyst for enzymatic reactions. A deficiency of this element can disrupt reactions and processes, causing harmful health effects.

Paul BT, Manz DH, Torti FM, Torti SV. **Mitochondria and Iron: current questions.** Expert Rev Hematol. 2017 Jan;10(1):65-79. doi: 10.1080/17474086.2016.1268047. Epub 2016 Dec 12. Erratum in: Expert Rev Hematol. 2017 Mar;10(3):275. PMID: 27911100; PMCID: PMC5538026.

Extracellular iron acts in the mitochondria as a cofactor of enzymes involved in oxidation-reduction reactions, DNA synthesis and repair and a variety of other processes. Iron is also essential in the mitochondria for the final steps of haem synthesis.
Iron is part of the very important enzymes in the citric acid cycle and in obtaining ATP energy.

Isaac IS, Dawson JH. **Haem iron-containing pe-**

roxidases. Essays Biochem. 1999;34:51-69. doi: 10.1042/bse0340051. PMID: 10730188.

It protects cells against oxidative stress by supporting the action of enzymes that break down reactive oxygen species. Such enzymes include oxidase, peroxidase, and catalase.

It should also be remembered that excessive amounts of iron can create reactive oxygen species which lead to oxidative stress.

Arora NP, Ghali JK. **Iron deficiency anemia in heart failure**. Heart Fail Rev. 2013 Jul;18(4):485-501. doi: 10.1007/s10741-012-9342-y. PMID: 22948485.

Iron is involved in the production and differentiation of red blood cells. It is needed for the production of hemoglobin, a protein found in red blood cells that is essential for the transport of oxygen around the body.

Arora NP, Ghali JK. **Iron deficiency anemia in heart failure.** Heart Fail Rev. 2013 Jul;18(4):485-501. doi: 10.1007/s10741-012-9342-y. PMID: 22948485.

As a component of myoglobin, it transports oxygen to the muscles. Myoglobin is a protein involved in the storage of oxygen in the red muscles.

Lozoff B. **Early iron deficiency has brain and behavior effects consistent with dopaminergic dysfunction.** J Nutr. 2011;141(4):740S-746S. doi:10.3945/jn.110.131169

"Iron deficiency also has other effects, specifically on other neurotransmitters, myelination, dendritogenesis, neurometabolism in hippocampus and striatum, gene and protein profiles, and associated behaviors. The persistence of poorer cognitive, motor, affective, and sensory system functioning highlights the need to prevent iron deficiency in infancy and to find interventions that lessen the long-term effects of this widespread nutrient disorder."

Iron is involved in the synthesis of neurotransmitters and myelin in the brain. Therefore, iron deficiency can have a negative impact on cognition in humans.

Iron is involved in the production and degradation of DNA, RNA, proteins, carbohydrates and lipids.

Iron deficiency can exist with or without anemia. Iron deficiency is also associated with weakened immunity. In the case of iron deficiency during pregnancy, both mother and baby can experience negative effects. Deficiencies increase risk of sepsis, maternal mortality, perinatal mortality, and low birth weight.

Lieu PT, Heiskala M, Peterson PA, Yang Y. **The roles of iron in health and disease.** Mol Aspects Med. 2001 Feb-Apr;22(1-2):1-87. doi: 10.1016/s0098-2997(00)00006-6. PMID: 11207374.

Iron deficiency can lead to fatigue.

Vaucher P, Druais PL, Waldvogel S, Favrat B. **Effect of iron supplementation on fatigue in nonanemic menstruating women with low ferritin:** a randomized controlled trial. CMAJ. 2012;184(11):1247-1254. doi:10.1503/cmaj.110950

"We found that iron supplementation for 12 weeks decreased fatigue by almost 50% from baseline (...)"
Iron supplementation significantly reduced fatigue in women with iron deficiency.

Ericsson, P. (1970), **THE EFFECT OF IRON SUPPLEMENTATION ON THE PHYSICAL WORK CAPACITY IN THE ELDERLY.** Acta Medica Scandinavica, 188: 361-374. https: //doi. org/10.1111/j. 0954-6820.1970.tb08052.x

In the case of apparently healthy men and women

of ages 58–71 years, iron supplementation increased exercise capacity in men by 4% and in women
by 12%.

Iron deficiency is associated with autism and poor
cognitive and social development in children.

Chocano-Bedoya PO, Manson JE, Hankinson SE,
et al. **Intake of selected minerals and risk
of premenstrual syndrome.** Am J Epidemiol.
2013;177(10):1118-1127. doi:10.1093/aje/kws363

Iron deficiency increases the risk of premenstrual
syndrome and women who get more than the recommended daily amount of iron may be less likely
to get a more severe form of PMS.

Khatiwada, S., Gelal, B., Baral, N. et al. **Association
between iron status and thyroid function in Nepa-
lese children.** Thyroid Res 9, 2 (2016). https: //doi.
org/10.1186/s13044-016-0031-0

"Thus, anemia and iron deficiency seems to be
associated with thyroid dysfunction particularly
hypothyroidism."
Iron deficiency impairs thyroid function.

Iron deficiency is also associated with diseases

such as rheumatoid arthritis, inflammatory bowel disease and celiac disease.

Almost 60% of iron in the body is attached to hemoglobin, 10% to muscle myoglobin. and another 10% of iron is present in iron-containing enzymes. Approx. 20% is stored in proteins that store iron in cells. The liver has the greatest capacity to store excess iron.

Iron exists in heme and non-heme form.

Heme iron can be directly absorbed by intestinal cells, independent of gastric acidity and absorption inhibitors such as polyphenols. Moreover, heme iron is absorbed by almost 22%. It is found mainly in animal products.

Geisser P, Burckhardt S. **The pharmacokinetics and pharmacodynamics of iron preparations.** Pharmaceutics. 2011;3(1):12-33. Published 2011 Jan 4. doi:10.3390/pharmaceu-tics3010012

Non-heme iron is much more difficult to absorb than heme iron. In order for this form of iron to be absorbed effectively, there must be an adequate acidic environment in the stomach. Non-heme iron is absorbed only in 2–5%.

Interestingly, most of the iron is obtained by recovering the iron from red blood cells.

Approximately 1-2 mg of iron is lost through sweat and blood each day. As there is also no pathway for iron excretion from the body, iron levels are regulated by increasing or decreasing iron absorption in the small intestine.

Daily iron requirements:

Men (19–70 years) - 8 mg

Women (19 - 50 years old) - 18 mg

Pregnant women - 27 mg

It is not a mineral that should be added without prior need, as determined by a doctor.

Food rich in iron in mg/100g:

- Chicken Liver - 12
- Dark chocolate - 10
- Pumpkin Seeds - 3.3
- Cashew nuts - 6.1
- Spinach - 2.7

IODINE

This is one of the elements with which there is the most misunderstanding. Iodine receptors are found on every cell in our body. Organs such as the gastric mucosa, breasts and salivary glands store a similar amount of iodine as the thyroid gland. Iodine is also needed by the ovaries, thymus, prostate, skin, joints, brain, arteries and bones.

The safe form of iodine is iodine in an inorganic and non-radioactive form. Only.

The Safe and Effective Implementation of Orthoiodosupplementation In Medical Practice Guy. E. Abraham M. D

Three generations of physicians have shown that administration in the form of iodine / potassium iodide in amounts of 12.5 to 37.6 mg is completely safe.

Orthoiodosupplementation in a Primary Care Practice
Jorge D. Flechas, M. D

Dr. Guy Abraham, Dr. Fleches and Dr. Brownstein, based on many years of experience, have found that the actual body's need for iodine is met by a dose of 12.5 mg per day. Nowadays the recommended daily limit for iodine intake is 150 micrograms for men and non-pregnant women. That's over 80 times less! Their research included 4,000 people who took 12.5 mg of iodine daily, and up to 100 mg of iodine daily in diabetics. These doses completely healed the breast lumps and the diabetic patients used less insulin. Many patients also got rid of migraines.

Thyroid function remained unchanged in 99% of patients. Side effects were less than 1% of patients. Often, excess iodine combined with a metallic aftertaste or acne has been associated with the bromine removal process. It resolved after dose reduction. "After treating over 1,000 patients with iodine, I have at no time seen the Wolff-Chaikoff Effect."

Kelly FC. **Iodine in Medicine and Pharmacy Since its Discovery**-1811-1961. Proc R Soc Med. 1961;54 (10): 1961;54 (10):831-836.

Despite the great fear of iodine, which is now commonplace, as early as 1956 there were 1,700 iodine-containing preparations with thousands of evidence demonstrating their efficacy and safety.

Wartofsky L, Ransil BJ, Ingbar SH. **Inhibition by iodine of the release of thyroxine from the thyroid glands of patients with thyrotoxicosis.** J Clin Invest. 1970 Jan;49(1):78-86. doi: 10.1172/JCI106225. PMID: 5409810; PMCID: PMC322446.

In 1970, the effects of Lugol's solution were evaluated by administering it to humans in an amount of 30 mg three times a day. In hyperthyroidism, the iodine / iodide contained in Lugol's solution administered in a daily dose of 90 mg causes a physiological tendency towards the normalization of thyroid function.

The Wolff-Chaikoff effect turned out to be a hoax.

Iodine affects the hormonal balance. Especially it concerns women and the estrogens they produce. Hormone imbalance can lead to cancer.

Dr. Jonathan Wright has shown that iodine in the form of Lugol's solution helps to keep estrogens in the correct proportions. He also showed that Lugol's solution favors the production of estriol (one of three estrogens: estrone, estradiol and estriol), which prevents the formation of cancer.

Maintaining a proper estrogen balance is almost impossible with iodine deficiency.

Stadel BV. **Dietary iodine and risk of**

breast, endometrial, and ovarian cancer. Lancet. 1976 Apr 24;1(7965):890-1. doi: 10.1016/s0140-6736(76)92102-4. PMID: 58152.

Venturi S, Donati FM, Venturi A, Venturi M, Grossi L, Guidi A. **Role of iodine in evolution and carcinogenesis of thyroid, breast and stomach**. Adv Clin Path. 2000 Jan;4(1):11-7. PMID: 10936894.

American specialists working with iodine agree that with iodine deficiency there is an increased incidence of breast, stomach, thyroid, ovarian, uterine and esophageal cancers. Therefore, special attention should be paid to iodine in cancer as it can help a lot in treatment.

Smyth, P.P.A. **Thyroid Disease and Breast Cancer**. J Endocrinol Invest 16, 396–401 (1993). https://doi.org/10.1007/BF03348865

Hypothyroidism promotes decreased immunity in the whole organism. Women with this disease are more likely to develop breast cancer.

The immunity-supporting effect does not only apply to cancer, of course. In the event of any infection, be it bacterial or viral, we should also take care of iodine. In very severe conditions (eg of

Covid-19), administration of 50 to 100 mg of iodine for two or three days and then 25 mg per day may prove very beneficial in the patient's treatment.

Jorge D. Flechas, M.D. treated patients with fibrocystic breast disease (FBD) with iodine doses ranging from 12.5 mg to 50 mg (4 tablets of Iodoral ®). Patients' breast pain disappeared within 1-30 days with the use of 50 mg of iodine. With lower iodine doses, this time was longer. When the ailment subsided, the doctor recommended taking 12.5-25 mg of iodine daily.

Iodine may prove useful in the treatment of diabetes. The same doctor, using 50 mg of iodine, made the patients able to significantly reduce the amount of insulin needed.

The same amounts of iodine per day can lead to cysts disappearance and return to normal period in patients with polycystic ovarian syndrome (PCOS).

Iodine is very important in the development of the fetus.

Hetzel BS. **Iodine and neuropsychological development.** J Nutr. 2000 Feb;130(2S Suppl):493S-495S. doi: 10.1093/jn/130.2.493S. PMID: 10721937.

Low iodine intake can adversely affect a child's physical and cognitive development. In extreme cases, congenital hypothyroidism occurs, which results in cretinism. Moderate iodine deficiency in pregnant women causes abnormalities in the intellectual development of the future baby.

Tiwari BD, Godbole MM, Chattopadhyay N, Mandal A, Mithal A. **Learning disabilities and poor motivation to achieve due to prolonged iodine deficiency.** Am J Clin Nutr. 1996 May;63(5):782-6. doi: 10.1093/ajcn/63.5.782. PMID: 8615364.

A meta-analysis indicates that iodine deficiency was the cause of of lower IQ in children.

Bleichrodt N, Shrestha RM, West CE, Hautvast JG, van de Vijver FJ, Born MP. **The benefits of adequate iodine intake.** Nutr Rev. 1996 Apr;54(4 Pt 2):S72-8. doi: 10.1111/j.1753-4887.1996.tb03901.x. PMID: 8700456.

Iodine deficiencies are associated with congenital defects, miscarriages or stillbirth. In addition, women with iodine deficiency who are breastfeeding may have difficulty making sure their baby receives the right amount of iodine in the milk.

van den Briel T, West CE, Bleichrodt N, van de Vijver FJ, Ategbo EA, Hautvast JG. **Improved iodine status is associated with improved mental performance of schoolchildren in Benin.** Am J Clin Nutr. 2000 Nov;72(5):1179-85. doi: 10.1093/ajcn/72.5.1179. PMID: 11063446.

"Children with increased urinary iodine concentrations had a significantly greater increase in performance on the combination of mental tests than did the group with no change in urinary iodine concentrations."

A study looking at the effects of iodized salt and other types of iodine supplements among children in Africa found that children taking iodine outperformed children with low iodine levels.

Zimmermann MB, Adou P, Torresani T, Zeder C, Hurrell RF. **Effect of oral iodized oil on thyroid size and thyroid hormone metabolism in children with concurrent selenium and iodine deficiency.** Eur J Clin Nutr. 2000 Mar;54(3):209-13. doi: 10.1038/sj.ejcn.1600921. PMID: 10713742.

Selenium deficiency makes children less responsive to iodine supplements, so it's important to consider your selenium intake as well.

Starr P, Walcott HP, Segall HN, et al. **The effect of iodine in exophthalmic goiter.** Atl Med J, 1924; 34:355-364

THOMPSON WO, THOMPSON PK, BRAILEY AG, COHEN AC. **PROLONGED TREATMENT OF EXOPH-THALMIC GOITER BY IODINE ALONE.** Arch Intern Med (Chic). 1930;45(4):481–502. doi:10.1001/archinte.1930.00140100003001

By using only iodine, 88% of patients with hyperthyroidism were cured. Other doctors using regular Lugol's solution achieved a cure in 92% of cases with a dose of 6-90 mg. There were no side effects.

Von Basedow GA. **Exophthalmos durch Hyperrophie des Zellgewebca in der Augenhöhle.** Wsrchr Ges Heilk, 1840; 6:197

Iodine was used as early as 1840 in the treatment of Graves' disease by von Besedow himself.

THOMPSON WO, THOMPSON PK, BRAILEY AG, COHEN AC. **PROLONGED TREATMENT OF EXOPH-THALMIC GOITER BY IODINE ALONE.** Arch Intern Med (Chic). 1930;45(4):481–502. doi:10.1001/archinte.1930.00140100003001

Other doctors have also treated Graves' disease.

Abraham, G.. "The Safe and Effective Implementation of Orthoiodosupplementation In Medical Practice." (2015).

"Of all the elements known so far to be essential for health, iodine is the most misunderstood and the most feared. Yet, it is by far the safest of all the trace elements known to be essential for human health. It is the only trace element that can be ingested safely in amounts up to 100,000 times the RDA. For example, potassium iodide has been prescribed safely to pulmonary patients in daily amounts of up to 6.0 gm/day, in large groups of such patients for several years. It is important, however, to emphasize that this safety record only applies to inorganic, non-radioactive iodine/iodide, not to organic iodine-containing drugs and to radioiodides. Unfortunately, the severe side effects of iodine-containing drugs have been attributed to inorganic iodine/iodide, even though published studies clearly demonstrate that it is the whole organic molecule that is cytotoxic, not the iodine covalently bound to this molecule."

In the above study, Dr. Abraham also shows the results of "Effect of Supplementation with a Complete Nutritional Program Combined with Iodine/Iodide at 12,5 mg/day on Thyroid Function Tests in a 40-year-old Female Patient with Graves'-Disease"

Zimmermann MB, Aeberli I, Melse-Boonstra A, Grimci L, Bridson J, Chaouki N, Mbhenyane X, Jooste PL. **Iodine treatment in children with subclinical hypothyroidism due to chronic iodine deficiency decreases thyrotropin and C-peptide concentrations and improves the lipid profile.** Thyroid. 2009 Oct;19(10):1099-104. doi: 10.1089/thy.2009.0001. PMID: 19534625.

In children with mild iodine deficiency, iodine supplementation lowered both markers of inflammation and cholesterol.

Iodine is extremely effective against bacteria, mold, yeast, protozoa and viruses. Iodine kills about 90% of the bacteria on the skin within 90 seconds. Moreover, it does not make bacteria resistant like antibiotics do.

Proper iodine supplementation shows increased removal of toxins in the urine.
When using three tablets of Iodoral ® (5 mg of iodine and 7.5 mg of potassium iodide) in the urine of people who took them, 20 times more compounds of bromine and fluoride appeared. The body also got rid of substances such as mercury, cadmium, arsenic and aluminum.

Iodized salt is not the best source of iodine.

In the case of supplementation, you should also take care of selenium, magnesium, copper, but also vitamin B2 and B3. This should be done in collaboration with a good endocrinologist.

CHROMIUM

Chromium is an essential mineral. It is essential that it is safe for consumption, i.e. trivalent chromium. Hexavalent chromium is toxic and carcinogenic.

Chromium is a cofactor of many important enzymes and increases the activity of the enzyme catalase (CAT), for example.

It can be very helpful in diabetes, especially as we now have an epidemic of this disease. It turns out 34.2 million Americans have diabetes and 88 million American adults are prediabetic (approximately 1 in 3). Can anything be done about it? Yes, and I have already written a bit about that. This element may also be important.

Anderson RA. **Chromium in the prevention and control of diabetes.** Diabetes Metab. 2000 Feb;26(1):22-7. PMID: 10705100.

Chromium increases the activity of insulin receptors and the uptake of insulin by cells. It leads to increased insulin sensitivity. This is crucial and applies to people with both type 1 and 2 diabetes.

Martin J, Wang ZQ, Zhang XH, Wachtel D, Volaufova J, Matthews DE, Cefalu WT. **Chromium picolinate supplementation attenuates body weight gain and increases insulin sensitivity in subjects with type 2 diabetes.** Diabetes Care. 2006 Aug;29(8):1826-32. doi: 10.2337/dc06-0254. PMID: 16873787.

Researchers at the University of Vermont also found that 1,000 μg of chromium picolinate administered for 6 months improved insulin sensitivity and glucose control in subjects with type 2 diabetes. Moreover, they proved that: "Further, CrPic supplementation significantly attenuated body weight gain and visceral fat accumulation compared with the placebo group."

Rabinovitz H, Friedensohn A, Leibovitz A, Gabay G, Rocas C, Habot B. **Effect of chromium supplementation on blood glucose and lipid levels in type 2 diabetes mellitus elderly patients.** Int J Vitam Nutr Res. 2004 May;74(3):178-82. doi: 10.1024/0300-9831.74.3.178. PMID: 15296075.

In the elderly group with type 2 diabetes, supplements helped control blood sugar levels and lower plasma lipid levels too.

Yanni AE, Stamataki NS, Konstantopoulos P, Stoupaki M, Abeliatis A, Nikolakea I, Perrea D, Karathanos VT, Tentolouris N. **Controlling type-2 diabetes by inclusion of Cr-enriched yeast bread in the daily dietary pattern:** a randomized clinical trial. Eur J Nutr. 2018 Feb;57(1):259-267. doi: 10.1007/s00394-016-1315-9. Epub 2016 Oct 12. PMID: 27734127.

Chromium enriched yeast supplementation to whole wheat bread in patients with type 2 diabetes "resulted in improvement of glucose tolerance and insulin resistance (...)". In addition, there was also a weight loss, a significant reduction in glycosylated hemoglobin and a lower systolic blood pressure.

Crawford V, Scheckenbach R, Preuss HG. **Effects of niacin-bound chromium supplementation on body composition in overweight African-American women.** Diabetes Obes Metab. 1999 Nov;1(6):331-7. doi: 10.1046/j.1463-1326.1999.00055.x. PMID: 11225649.

Niacin-bound chromium ingested daily over 2 months by African-American women caused a significant fat loss in conjunction with modest dietary and exercise regimen.

Chromium supports brain function

Krikorian R, Eliassen JC, Boespflug EL, Nash TA, Shidler MD. **Improved cognitive-cerebral function in older adults with chromium supplementation**. Nutr Neurosci. 2010 Jun;13(3):116-22. doi: 10.1179/147683010X12611460764084. PMID: 20423560.

A study in older adults found that chromium supplementation can improve memory. The study concerned people at risk of cognitive decline.
In addition, chromium supplementation may help with depression in some respects.

Jin Y, Liu L, Zhang S, Tao B, Tao R, He X, Qu L, Huang J, Wang X, Fu Z. **Chromium alters lipopolysaccharide-induced inflammatory responses both in vivo and in vitro.** Chemosphere. 2016 Apr;148:436-43. doi: 10.1016/j.chemosphere.2016.01.057. Epub 2016 Feb 4. PMID: 26841286.

Administration of chromium in mice decreased the inflammatory response, demonstrating its anti-inflammatory properties.

It affects bone health.

McCarty MF. **Anabolic effects of insulin on bone suggest a role for chromium pi-**

colinate in preservation of bone density. Med Hypotheses. 1995 Sep;45(3):241-6. doi: 10.1016/0306-9877(95)90112-4. PMID: 8569546.

In postmenopausal women, supplementation with chromium picolinate reduces bone resorption, which may play a vital role in the preservation of postmenopausal bone density.

Jamilian M, Bahmani F, Siavashani MA, Mazloomi M, Asemi Z, Esmaillzadeh A. **The Effects of Chromium Supplementation on Endocrine Profiles, Biomarkers of Inflammation, and Oxidative Stress in Women with Polycystic Ovary Syndrome:** a Randomized, Double-Blind, Placebo-Controlled Trial. Biol Trace Elem Res. 2016 Jul;172(1):72-78. doi: 10.1007/s12011-015-0570-6. Epub 2015 Nov 28. PMID: 26613790.

In women with polycystic ovary syndrome, chromium supplementation lowers the levels of proteins associated with heart disease, improves skin lesions, and increases the body's ability to deal with free radicals.

Determining the level of chromium is especially important for diabetics.
The daily requirement of chromium for adults is 35

mcg for men and 25 mcg for women.
High chromium foods per 100g:
- Mussel 128 mcg
- Brazil nut 100 mcg
- Brown shrimp 26 mcg
- Tomato 20 mcg
- Broccoli 16 mcg
- Egg yolk 6 mcg
- Pear 26 mcg

MANGANESE

Manganese is a trace mineral, which your body needs in small amounts. It is an essential element for all living organisms. It acts as a cofactor for many important enzymes. Mitochondria are the organelles that are the richest in manganese. Both manganese deficiency and excess are toxic to the mitochondria. Excess, among other things, leads to the excessive production of radical oxygen species (ROS).

Manganese protects against oxidative and nitrosative stress. It is a cofactor of antioxidant enzymes.

Aguirre JD, Culotta VC. **Battles with iron: manganese in oxidative stress protection.** J Biol Chem. 2012;287(17):13541-13548. doi:10.1074/jbc.R111.312181

Thus, it prevents cell damage

Martinez-Finley EJ, Gavin CE, Aschner M, Gunter TE. **Manganese neurotoxicity and the role of reactive oxygen species.** Free Radic Biol Med. 2013;62:65-75. doi:10.1016/j.freeradbiomed.2013.01.032

Mn-dependent superoxide dismutase (MnSOD) neutralizes the toxic effects of reactive oxygen species (ROS) in the mitochondria.

Bu SY, Choi MK. **Daily Manganese Intake Status and Its Relationship with Oxidative Stress Biomarkers under Different Body Mass Index Categories in Korean Adults.** Clin Nutr Res. 2012;1(1):30-36. doi:10.7762/cnr.2012.1.1.30

"MnSOD is reported to protect cells from various carcinogens such as toxic chemical substances and radioactive materials, oxidative stresses and inflammatory responses."

Martinez-Finley EJ, Gavin CE, Aschner M, Gunter TE. **Manganese neurotoxicity and the role of reactive oxygen species.** Free Radic Biol Med. 2013;62:65-75. doi:10.1016/j.freeradbiomed.2013.01.032

The manganese-containing catalase enzyme is an essential enzyme that converts hydrogen peroxide and thus reduces oxidative stress.

Davis CD, Greger JL. **Longitudinal changes of**

manganese-dependent superoxide dismutase and other indexes of manganese and iron status in women. Am J Clin Nutr. 1992 Mar;55(3):747-52. doi: 10.1093/ajcn/55.3.747. PMID: 1550052.

In a study of 47 young women, oxidative stress was lower in women supplementing manganese.

Manganese may also be crucial in the metabolic syndrome, insulin resistance and diabetes.

Du S, Wu X, Han T, Duan W, Liu L, Qi J, Niu Y, Na L, Sun C. **Dietary manganese and type 2 diabetes mellitus**: two prospective cohort studies in China. Diabetologia. 2018 Sep;61(9):1985-1995. doi: 10.1007/s00125-018-4674-3. Epub 2018 Jul 3. PMID: 29971528.

A study of over 10,000 people found that higher dietary manganese intake was associated with a lower incidence of type 2 diabetes.

Hajra B, Orakzai BA, Faryal U, Hassan M, Rasheed S, Wazir S. **Insulin Sensitivity To Trace Metals (Chromium, Manganese) In Type 2 Diabetic Patients And Non Diabetic Individuals**. J Ayub Med Coll Abbottabad. 2016 Jul-Sep;28(3):534-536. PMID: 28712229.

"Low serum level of Chromium and manganese were found in diabetic patients as compare to non-diabetic individuals."

Research shows lower blood manganese levels in people with diabetes.

Manganese deficiency is associated with a higher risk of developing diabetes. Supplementing this element in the event of deficiency can prevent the development of this disease. However, an excess can have the opposite effect and you should be careful.

Li Y, Guo H, Wu M, Liu M. **Serum and dietary antioxidant status is associated with lower prevalence of the metabolic syndrome in a study in Shanghai, China**. Asia Pac J Clin Nutr. 2013;22(1):60-8. doi: 10.6133/apjcn.2013.22.1.06. PMID: 23353612.

A study with 221 cases and 329 controls aged 18 to 65 years showed that people with higher manganese levels had a significantly lower risk of metabolic syndrome.

Choi MK, Bae YJ. **Relationship between dietary magnesium, manganese, and copper and metabolic syndrome risk in Korean adults**: the Korea National Health and Nutrition Examination Survey (2007-2008). Biol Trace Elem

Res. 2013 Dec;156(1-3):56-66. doi: 10.1007/s12011-013-9852-z. Epub 2013 Nov 12. PMID: 24218228.

In addition, over 5,000 Korean adult women with metabolic syndrome have been shown to have lower daily manganese intake.
Higher manganese intake is also associated with lower triglyceride levels.

Haynes EN, Sucharew H, Kuhnell P, et al. **Manganese Exposure and Neurocognitive Outcomes in Rural School-Age Children:** The Communities Actively Researching Exposure Study (Ohio, USA). Environ Health Perspect. 2015;123(10):1066-1071. doi:10.1289/ehp.1408993

Low manganese levels are associated with lower IQ scores in children. It is related to manganese affecting the activity of several enzymes also important for the work of the brain.

Zhou T, Guo J, Zhang J, Xiao H, Qi X, Wu C, Chang X, Zhang Y, Liu Q, Zhou Z. **Sex-Specific Differences in Cognitive Abilities Associated with Childhood Cadmium and Manganese Exposures in School-Age Children: a Prospective Cohort Study**. Biol Trace Elem Res. 2020 Jan;193(1):89-99. doi: 10.1007/s12011-019-01703-9. Epub 2019 Apr 11.

PMID: 30977088.

Another study involving 296 school-age children found that children with higher levels of manganese in their urine had a higher IQ.

Here it is still important to remember that it is about the right level of manganese. Deficiency and excess are detrimental to the proper development of a child and an adult.

Children with autism also have lower manganese levels.

Burton NC, Guilarte TR. **Manganese neurotoxicity: lessons learned from longitudinal studies in nonhuman primates.** Environ Health Perspect. 2009;117(3):325-332. doi:10.1289/ehp.0800035

Manganese deficiency can result in higher levels of glutamate in the brain, which is linked to autism. Furthermore, mitochondrial dysfunction is a major feature of autism. And manganese is needed for mitochondria to function properly.

Crossgrove J, Zheng W. **Manganese toxicity upon overexposure.** NMR Biomed. 2004;17(8):544-553. doi:10.1002/nbm.931

Patients with epilepsy also have low manganese levels. Some research suggests that some symptoms may correlate with its low levels.

Du K, Liu M, Pan Y, Zhong X, Wei M. **Association of Serum Manganese Levels with Alzheimer's Disease and Mild Cognitive Impairment**: A Systematic Review and Meta-Analysis. Nutrients. 2017 Mar 3;9(3):231. doi: 10.3390/nu9030231. PMID: 28273828; PMCID: PMC5372894.

In Alzheimer's disease is no different when it comes to manganese levels. Again, patients with Alzheimer's disease have significantly reduced blood manganese levels. Therefore, a deficiency may be a risk factor for this disease.

Here, too, there may be a connection with the malfunctioning of the mitochondria.
This mineral can prove to be useful for depression.

Młyniec K, Gaweł M, Doboszewska U, Starowicz G, Pytka K, Davies CL, Budziszewska B. **Essential elements in depression and anxiety.** Part II. Pharmacol Rep. 2015 Apr;67(2):187-94. doi: 10.1016/j.pharep.2014.09.009. Epub 2014 Sep 27. PMID: 25712638.

Its low levels can contribute to the development of

depression.

Nakamura M, Miura A, Nagahata T, Shibata Y, Okada E, Ojima T. **Low Zinc, Copper, and Manganese Intake is Associated with Depression and Anxiety Symptoms in the Japanese Working Population**: Findings from the Eating Habit and Well-Being Study. Nutrients. 2019;11(4):847. Published 2019 Apr 15. doi:10.3390/nu11040847

"In addition, we observed an inverse association between manganese intake and depression."
A study in over 2,000 Japanese has found a link between low dietary manganese levels and a higher risk of depression.

Miyake Y, Tanaka K, Okubo H, Sasaki S, Furukawa S, Arakawa M. **Manganese intake is inversely associated with depressive symptoms during pregnancy in Japan**: Baseline data from the Kyushu Okinawa Maternal and Child Health Study. J Affect Disord. 2017 Mar 15;211:124-129. doi: 10.1016/j.jad.2017.01.016. Epub 2017 Jan 15. PMID: 28110159.

Similarly, in a study of 1,745 pregnant Japanese women: "The current cross-sectional study of Japanese women demonstrated higher manganese intake to be independently associated with a lower prevalence of depressive symptoms during pregnancy."

Samsel A, Seneff S. **Glyphosate, pathways to modern diseases III: Manganese, neurological diseases, and associated pathologies**. Surg Neurol Int. 2015;6:45. Published 2015 Mar 24. doi:10.4103/2152-7806.153876

Manganese deficiency can reduce male fertility because manganese is important for normal sperm motility.

Shamberger RJ. **Calcium, magnesium, and other elements in the red blood cells and hair of normals and patients with premenstrual syndrome**. Biol Trace Elem Res. 2003 Aug;94(2):123-9. doi: 10.1385/BTER:94:2:123. PMID: 12958403.

Lower dietary manganese levels exacerbated pain symptoms during PMS (premenstrual syndrome). Additionally, a study of 96 women with PMS also showed lower blood manganese levels.

Manganese is important for cartilage and bones. It is a component of various enzymes involved in the production of these parts. In addition, it plays a vital role in introducing calcium into the bones.

Manganese may also prove to be crucial in cancer prevention. The enzyme I mentioned before (MnSOD) is related to cancer prevention.

Shen F, Cai WS, Li JL, Feng Z, Cao J, Xu B. **The association between deficient manganese levels and breast cancer**: a meta-analysis. Int J Clin Exp Med. 2015;8(3):3671-3680. Published 2015 Mar 15.

"In conclusion, this meta-analysis supports a significant association between deficient Mn levels and breast cancer."
A meta-analysis of 11 studies involving 1,302 patients shows that women with breast cancer have lower levels of manganese than healthy women.

Farina M, Avila DS, da Rocha JB, Aschner M. **Metals, oxidative stress and neurodegeneration: a focus on iron, manganese and mercury.** Neurochem Int. 2013;62(5):575-594. doi:10.1016/j.neuint.2012.12.006

Up to about 11 mg of manganese per day, no side effects are observed. In the case of identified deficiencies, supplementation should be approx. 2 to 5 mg per day.
The body naturally regulates its absorption. If we eat a lot of manganese-rich foods, the body will ab-

sorb less manganese.

High manganese foods per 100g:
- Mussels (296% DV)
- Sweet Potatoes (43% DV)
- Firm Tofu (51% DV)
- Pine Nuts (383% DV) and 12 hazelnuts (70% DV)
- Brown Rice (48% DV)
- Spinach (41% DV)
- Pineapple (40% DV)

BORON

Boron appears to be very beneficial to our health and itself affects many biochemical processes in our body.

Boron can ameliorate or prevent arthritic symptoms.

Newnham, RE . **How boron is being used in medical practice**. In: Goldbach, HE, Rerkasem, B, Wimmer, MA, Brown, PH, Thellier, M, Bell, RW, eds. Boron in Plant and Animal Nutrition. New York, NY: Kluwer Academic/Plenum; 2002:59–62.

Newnham, based only on observations, found that the occurrence of arthritis is less where there is more boron in the water and soil.

Richard L. Travers, George C. Rennie & Rex E. Newnham (1990) **Boron and Arthritis**: The Results of a Double-blind Pilot Study, Journal of Nutritional Medicine, 1:2, 127-132, DOI: 10.3109/13590849009003147

In an Australian study of 20 osteoarthritis patients

who were given 6 mg of boron daily for 8 weeks: "Of the 10 patients on boron, five improved and five did not, but only one of the 10 patients on the placebo improved".

However, 5 people did not complete the study, so the condition improved in 71% (5/7) of those who took boron.

It also turned out that in patients with rheumatoid arthritis the level of boron, e.g. in the bones, was lower.

Miljkovic D, Scorei RI, Cimpoiaşu VM, Scorei ID. **Calcium fructoborate: plant-based dietary boron for human nutrition**. J Diet Suppl. 2009;6(3):211-26. doi: 10.1080/19390210903070772. PMID: 22435474.

In another study, boron supplementation also alleviated subjective measures of arthritis. The pain has also decreased.

Peng X, Lingxia Z, Schrauzer GN, Xiong G. **Selenium, boron, and germanium deficiency in the etiology of Kashin-Beck disease**. Biol Trace Elem Res. 2000 Dec;77(3):193-7. doi: 10.1385/BTER:77:3:193. PMID: 11204461.

A disorder of the bones and joints Kashin-Beck disease can also be associated with a boron deficiency. Boron deficiency and increased parathyroid hormone level causes also bone decalcification. Higher levels of calcium in the blood lead to degeneration and inflammation of the joints as well as osteoporosis. After some time, soft tissue calcification and kidney stones may also develop.

Boron can affect the immune system.

Bai, Y, Hunt, CD, Newman, SM. **Dietary boron increases serum antibody (IgG and IgM) concentrations in rats immunized with human typhoid vaccine.** Proc N D Acad Sci. 1997;51:81.

Scientists showed that boron supplementation increased antibody concentrations in animals injected with antibody-inducing agents. They also stated that boron deficiency may diminish immune function.

Nielsen, FH, Penland, JG. **Boron supplementation of peri-menopausal women affects boron metabolism and indices associated with macromineral metabolism, hormonal status and immune function.** J Trace Elem Exp Med. 1999;12:251–261.

Boron supplementation in women significantly increased white blood cell numbers, increased percentage of neutrophils (a type of white blood cell that, inter alia, protect us from infections), and decreased percentage of lymphocytes.

Nielsen, FH. **Evidence for the nutritional essentiality of boron**. J Trace Elem Exp Med. 1996;9:215–229.

Boron supplementation at 3 mg per day significantly increased erythrocyte superoxide dismutase concentration (performing antioxidant functions) in people with boron deficiency (0.25 mg / d).
Boron turns out to be important for bone health.

Hunt CD, Herbel JL, Idso JP. **Dietary boron modifies the effects of vitamin D3 nutrition on indices of energy substrate utilization and mineral metabolism in the chick**. J Bone Miner Res. 1994 Feb;9(2):171-82. doi: 10.1002/jbmr.5650090206. PMID: 8140930.

Findings indicate that boron deprivation was detrimental to bone growth in chicks.

Nielsen FH, Stoecker BJ. **Boron and fish oil have different beneficial effects on strength and trabecular microarchitecture of bone**. J Trace Elem

Med Biol. 2009;23(3):195-203. doi: 10.1016/j.j-temb.2009.03.003. Epub 2009 May 8. PMID: 19486829.

"A three-point bending test for bone strength found that boron deprivation decreased the maximum force needed to break the femur."

Microcomputed tomography in rats has shown that the supply of boron is beneficial for trabecular bone microarchitecture.

Gorustovich AA, Steimetz T, Nielsen FH, Gugliel-motti MB. **Histomorphometric study of alveolar bone healing in rats fed a boron-deficient diet.** Anat Rec (Hoboken). 2008 Apr;291(4):441-7. doi: 10.1002/ar.20672. PMID: 18361451.

In a study on rats regarding bone healing after tooth extraction, scientists concluded: "The findings show that boron deficiency results in altered bone healing because of a marked reduction in osteogenesis".

Uysal T, Ustdal A, Sonmez MF, Ozturk F. **Stimulation of bone formation by dietary boron in an orthopedically expanded suture in rabbits.** Angle Orthod. 2009 Sep;79(5):984-90. doi: 10.2319/112708-604.1. PMID: 19705952.

In a study on rabbits, boron has been found to stimulate dental bone formation.

Scorei, R, Rotaru, P. **Calcium fructoborate: potential anti-inflammatory agent** [published online ahead of print January 28, 2011]. Biol Trace Elem Res. ;doi:10.1007/s12011-011-8972-6.

Calcium fructoborate in particular may be useful in the treatment of osteoporosis. Dietary boron supplementation improved bone density in 66 out of 100 osteoporosis patients.

Cui Y, Winton MI, Zhang ZF, Rainey C, Marshall J, De Kernion JB, Eckhert CD. **Dietary boron intake and prostate cancer risk**. Oncol Rep. 2004 Apr;11(4):887-92. PMID: 15010890.

Scientists speculated that there is an inverse association between dietary boron and prostate cancer.

Barranco WT, Eckhert CD. **Boric acid inhibits human prostate cancer cell proliferation.** Cancer Lett. 2004 Dec 8;216(1):21-9. doi: 10.1016/j.canlet.2004.06.001. PMID: 15500945.

Other scientists have found that boric acid inhibits

the proliferation (rapid reproduction) of prostate cancer cell lines. With dose-dependent amounts of boron, observations also indicated the presence of apoptosis.

The positive effect of boron may also apply to breast cancer.

Korkmaz M, Uzgören E, Bakirdere S, Aydin F, Ataman OY. **Effects of dietary boron on cervical cytopathology and on micronucleus frequency in exfoliated buccal cells.** Environ Toxicol. 2007 Feb;22(1):17-25. doi: 10.1002/tox.20229. PMID: 17295277.

Researchers took cervical smears from 1059 women. 472 of the women lived in relatively boron-rich (intake of boron was about 8.41 mg / day) rural areas. 587 of the women lived in relatively boron-poor (intake of boron was about 1.26 mg / day) areas. Women from regions with higher boron intake did not have cytopathological indications of cervical cancer. For women who consumed less boron, there were cytopathological findings for 15 women. The researchers concluded: "The results suggest that ingestion of boron in the drinking water decreases the incidence of cervical cancer-related histopathological findings".

Mahabir S, Spitz MR, Barrera SL, Dong YQ, Eastham C, Forman MR. **Dietary boron and hormone replacement therapy as risk factors for lung cancer in women.** Am J Epidemiol. 2008 May 1;167(9):1070-80. doi: 10.1093/aje/kwn021. Epub 2008 Mar 14. PMID: 18343880; PMCID: PMC3390773.

Another case-control study of 1,601 people revealed that boron intake was inversely associated with lung cancer.

Boron supports the work of the brain.

Penland JG. **The importance of boron nutrition for brain and psychological function.** Biol Trace Elem Res. 1998 Winter;66(1-3):299-317. doi: 10.1007/BF02783144. PMID: 10050926.

Research indicates that in the event of a boron deficiency, brain electrical activity is reduced. Boron deficiencies cause poorer performance on tasks of motor speed, short-term memory, dexterity and attention.

Penland JG. **Dietary boron, brain function, and cognitive performance.** Environ Health Perspect. 1994 Nov;102 Suppl 7(Suppl 7):65-72. doi: 10.1289/ehp.94102s765. PMID: 7889884; PMCID:

PMC1566632.

From an abstract from another scientific publication:

"Performance (e.g., response time) on various cognitive and psy-chomotor tasks also showed an effect of dietary boron. When contrasted with the high boron intake, low dietary boron resulted in significantly poorer performance ($p < 0.05$) on tasks emphasizing manual dexterity (studies II and III); eye-hand coordination (study II); attention (all studies); perception (study III); encoding and short-term memory (all studies); and long-term memory (study I). Collectively, the data from these three studies indicate that boron may play a role in human brain function and cognitive performance, and provide additional evidence that boron is an essential nutrient for humans".

Boron affects the action of hormones such as estrogen, thyroid hormone, insulin, vitamin D and progesterone.

Nielsen, FH . **Evidence for the nutritional essentiality of boron**. J Trace Elem Exp Med. 1996;9:215–229.

In the case of boron supplementation in elderly people with boron deficiency in the amount of 3 mg a day, after 63 days, the level of vitamin D increased.

When rats were fed a highly oxidative diet, the additional amount of boron (from 0.4 mg / kg to 5 mg / kg) significantly increased the beneficial effect of estradiol supplementation.

We can conclude that boron may play an important role in the endocrine system of women.

Insufficient evidence suggests that boron may also have an effect on insulin action.

It is worth consuming products rich in boron, such as nuts or avocados.

Kuru R, Yilmaz S, Balan G, Tuzuner BA, Tasli PN, Akyuz S, Yener Ozturk F, Altuntas Y, Yarat A, Sahin F. **Boron-rich diet may regulate blood lipid profile and prevent obesity**: A non-drug and self-controlled clinical trial. J Trace Elem Med Biol. 2019 Jul;54:191-198. doi: 10.1016/j.jtemb.2019.04.021. Epub 2019 May 1. PMID: 31109611.

Thirteen healthy women consumed 10 mg more boron with boron-rich foods for one month then during their routine diet. There was a significant reduction in LDL, VLDL cholesterol, and triglyceride levels. Body Mass Index and body fat weight also decreased. Increased boron intake through dietary may have beneficial effects on lipid metabolism, obesity, and thyroid metabolism. The final positive effect may also be influenced by other substances found in the boron-rich foods.

The daily boron intake should definitely not be less than 3 mg per day. The upper limit is difficult to define at the stage of the knowledge we have. Rather and better not to exceed 30 mg of boron per day.

Food rich in boron in mg/100g:
- Almonds - 2.82
- Peanut Butter - 1.92
- Brazil Nuts - 1.72
- Walnut - 1.63
- Beans (kidney red) - 1,4
- Celery - 0.5
- Broccoli - 0.31 and carrot - 0.3

A FEW WORDS
AT THE END...

Any reasonably intelligent person after reading this book can come to at least one conclusion - to ensure health, we must take care of all vitamins and minerals. Of course, also proteins, fatty acids, etc... I consider the readers of this book to be intelligent people. The state of health in the world is poor. Knowledge about these topics too. And dietary recommendations are often at least idiotic. There are more and more patients and the therapies that have been used for decades by some doctors are forbidden. While medicine can cope with emergencies, operations, etc., it cannot cope with the treatment of autoimmune diseases or cancer, allegedly incurable diseases. As it turns out, incurable diseases are often curable. Some easier and some harder. What are we left to do? I think to make people aware and spread knowledge. Make doctors aware as well. I hope that in the future people will try to prevent the disease more and that doctors will be able to treat people more effectively. There is enough knowledge to do so...

Made in the USA
Monee, IL
06 April 2022

94254066R00125